Aids to Undergraduate Obstetrics and Gynaecology

For Churchill Livingstone

Publisher: Timothy Horne
Project Editor: Dilys Jones
Copy Editor: Susan Beasley
Indexer: J. Roderick Gibb
Production Controller: P.S.D.
Sales Promotion Executive: Marion Pollock

Aids to Undergraduate Obstetrics and Gynaecology

Christopher Sinclair
MB BS BSc

Senior Registrar in Public Health Medicine,
South West Thames Regional Health Authority;
formerly Senior House Officer in Obstetrics,
Northwick Park Hospital, London

J. Beverley Webb
FRCS MRCOG

Consultant Obstetrician and Gynaecologist,
Lister Hospital, Stevenage, Herts

SECOND EDITION

CHURCHILL LIVINGSTONE
EDINBURGH LONDON MADRID MELBOURNE NEW YORK AND TOKYO 1993

CHURCHILL LIVINGSTONE
Medical Division of Longman Group UK Limited

Distributed in the United States of America by Churchill
Livingstone Inc., 650 Avenue of the Americas, New York,
N.Y. 10011, and by associated companies, branches and
representatives throughout the world.

First edition 1986
Second edition 1993

ISBN 0-443-04785-5

British Library Cataloguing in Publication Data
A catalogue record for this book is available from the British
Library.

Library of Congress Cataloging in Publication Data
A catalog record for this book is available from the Library of
Congress.

The
publisher's
policy is to use
**paper manufactured
from sustainable forests**

Produced by Longman Publishers Singapore Pte Ltd
Printed in Singapore

Contents

Preface

This book is intended to enable the undergraduate to revise quickly and easily, by means of lists, the subject of Obstetrics and Gynaecology. The lists will jog the memory and aid recall of detail relating to the subject under revision. It is hoped that this will be of benefit in preparing for MCQs and written examinations. In addition some of the lists will provide ready-made essay plans.

The authors believe that examination technique is as important as adequate factual knowledge. When writing an essay, a plan must be constructed, and time left at the end for reading through, correction, and the underlining of important points which the candidate wishes to highlight to the examiner. The plans may be drawn up singly as each essay is tackled, or the first part of the examination may be allotted to planning all the essays, but whichever system is adopted, accurate time-keeping throughout is essential. It is worth noting that the candidate will often find that while preparing the second plan, ideas for the first will enter the mind, and that while writing the first essay, ideas for the last plan will interrupt the planned flow of thought. For this reason the second system is usually better.

We have not suggested a reading list or provided references since most undergraduates find their own books with a style that suits them. Nonetheless, we encourage the student to research further any points encountered with which he/she is not familiar, and more importantly, get to know the practices and their rationale in your teaching hospital. This will give you the ability and confidence to discuss them in a viva where you may well encounter external examiners who hold differing views to those you have been taught, e.g. the induction of labour. Do not worry; the internal examiner is there to see fair play and all that is expected of you is to prove that you are safe to be allowed to practise. Provided you achieve this, there is no reason why you should not succeed in passing your final examinations.

London and Stevenage, 1993

Acknowledgements

The authors would like to express their gratitude to Mrs Joyce Webb and Miss Julie Pollicott for typing the manuscripts, and to Churchill Livingstone for their tolerance and helpful guidance in the preparation of this book.

PART 1

Reproductive anatomy and physiology

Reproductive anatomy and physiology

This chapter outlines key anatomical and physiological facts, knowledge of which simplifies the understanding of clinical obstetrics and gynaecology. The selection has been made partly on the basis of clinical relevance and partly on the degree of interest shown in the matter by examiners.

MATERNAL AND GYNAECOLOGICAL ANATOMY

The bony pelvis
The bony pelvis provides the basic framework of the birth canal: for this reason its shape, size and clinically identifiable landmarks should be understood.

The pelvic diameters
In the past cephalo-pelvic disproportion (disparity between the size and shape of the fetal head and the maternal birth canal) accounted for a large proportion of difficult and obstructed labours. This resulted in the obstetrician's classical interest in pelvic dimensions. Figure 1 defines the key diameters.

Note that there is a 'pattern' to these measurements.

Pelvic shape
The pelvic inlet (brim) is bean-shaped with its greatest diameter placed transversely: hence the antero posterior (AP) diameter of the fetal head usually enters the pelvis in the transverse diameter.

The mid-cavity is roughly cylindrical to allow rotation of the presenting part and shoulders, and, in breech presentations, the after-coming head.

The outlet is diamond-shaped with its greatest diameter placed antero posteriorly: the fetal head leaves the pelvis with the sagittal suture in the AP diameter of the pelvic outlet. The axis of the outlet is at 90° to the axis of the inlet.

3

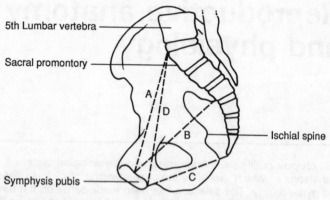

Fig. 1 Side view of the bony pelvis showing key diameters: for typical measurements see Table 1. A = pelvic inlet (brim); B = mid-cavity; C = pelvic outlet; D = diagonal (obstetric) conjugate

Table 1. Average dimensions of the bony pelvis (cm)

	Anteroposterior	Oblique	Transverse
Inlet	11	12	13
Mid-cavity	12	12	12
Outlet	13	12	11

The rotation of the fetal head during its passage through the pelvis is one of the key events in labour: failure to rotate, for example, may result in 'deep transverse arrest'.

Pelvic Landmarks

Sacral promontory: Palpation of this on vaginal examination suggests a short diagonal (obstetric) conjugate and therefore a small pelvis.

Ischial spines: These provide useful landmarks on the side of the birth canal to assess the descent of the presenting part.

Pubic arch:

Intertuberous }   These provide a crude assessment of pelvic outlet dimensions.
diameter

The method of palpating these landmarks is shown in Figure 2.

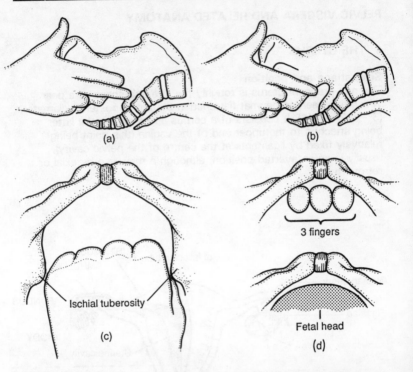

Fig. 2 (a) Attempting to palpate the sacral promontory; (b) palpating the ischial spine; (c) assessment of the intertuberous diameter; (d) assessment of the sub-pubic arch. *Note*: If the sub-pubic arch is narrow, the fetal head is pushed posteriorly, the 'dead space' is greater and the *effective* anterior posterior diameter of the outlet is reduced.

The pelvic floor

The pelvic floor (or diaphragm) is composed of muscles and condensations of fascia, perforated in three places by the urethra, vagina and anus. It performs a number of important functions including:

1. Support of the pelvic (and abdominal) viscera
2. Maintenance of continence (urinary and faecal)
3. Assisting in the rotation of the fetal head during labour.

It may be damaged in labour by stretching and denervation and subsequently fail to perform its functions, especially those of support and the maintenance of urinary continence.

PELVIC VISCERA AND RELATED ANATOMY

1. THE UTERUS

Size, shape and position
The non-pregnant uterus is roughly the size and shape of a pear which has been somewhat flattened in the anteroposterior diameter, ($3'' \times 2'' \times 1''$). It consists of a corpus and a cervix, the latter being attached to the upper end of the vagina (this point being relatively fixed by ligaments at the centre of the pelvic cavity), usually in an anteverted position, although it may also be axial or retroverted.

(a)

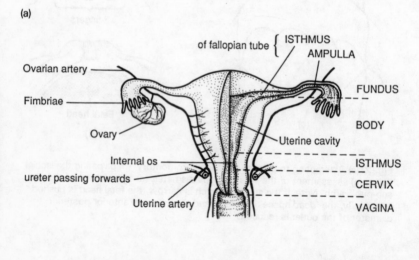

(b)

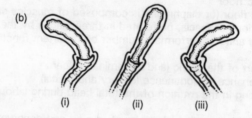

Fig. 3 (a) Anatomy of the uterus and (b) orientation of the uterus in (i) anteversion; (ii) axial position and (iii) retroversion

During pregnancy the uterus undergoes great enlargement, becoming palpable abdominally at about 12–14 weeks' gestation; thereafter it continues to grow as shown.

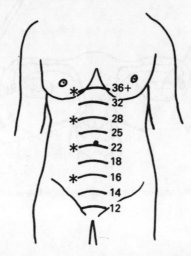

Fig. 4 Usual height of the uterine fundus at different weeks of gestation. Those levels marked * represent key dates which can usefully be learnt to allow extrapolation to other dates. Uterine size can also be assessed using a tape measure (pubic synthesis → fundus in centimetres = gestation in weeks ±2)

Blood supply and lymphatics

Blood supply: Mainly from the uterine artery which arises from the internal iliac artery, and subsequently anastomoses with the ovarian artery in the broad ligament. Just before reaching the uterus (at the level of the internal os) it crosses over the ureter, so exposing the latter to risk at hysterectomy. (Aide memoire: water under bridge).

Lymphatics: Clinically highly relevant because of metastatic spread from carcinoma. Note that the main drainage channels for the uterine body and uterine cervix follow different routes (the respective carcinomas also differ in their propensity to lymphatic spread).

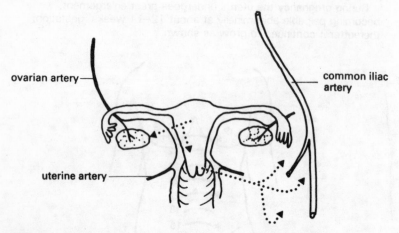

Fig. 5 Lymphatic drainage of the uterus; drainage follows the direction of the dotted lines

Ligaments

The main 'structural' ligaments which hold the uterus in place are attached to the cervix, from which they radiate out to become attached to various structures as shown in Figure 6.

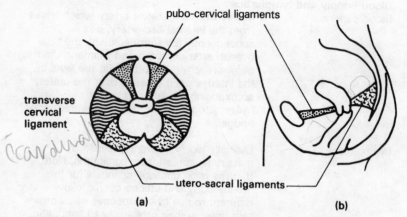

Fig. 6 The ligaments of the uterine cervix (a) as seen from below and (b) lateral view

The broad ligament

[handwritten: Uterus → side wall of pelvis]

This is not a true ligament but a fold of peritoneum draped over the fallopian tubes stretching from the lateral wall of the uterus to the side walls of the pelvis. (Anteriorly the peritoneum sweeps off the anterior uterus over the bladder forming the utero-vesical pouch. Posteriorly the peritoneum sweeps down the back of the uterus, cervix and posterior fornix of the vagina onto the anterior rectum forming the pouch of Douglas.)

The round ligament

[handwritten: upper uterus → internal inguinal ring → labius majus]

Represents the remains of the lower part of the gubernaculum and passes from the upper outer corner of the uterus to the internal inguinal ring, and from there to the labium majus. It is composed of smooth muscle and is greatly stretched in pregnancy, which may give rise to pain.

Congenital uterine anomalies

Four of the more common anomalies are illustrated (Fig. 7a–e). These often arise from abnormal development of the Wolffian and Muellerian ducts, and associated urinary tract abnormalities are common. IVU is recommended.

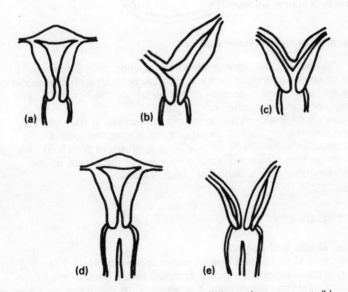

Fig. 7 Common congenital uterine anomalies: (a) normal arrangement; (b) rudimentary horn; (c) bicornuate uterus, normal vagina; (d) normal uterus with vaginal septum; (e) bicornuate uterus with septate vagina

Histology

The body of the uterus is lined internally by the endometrium, the innermost layer of which consists of columnar epithelium, which is invaginated to form the uterine glands. For this reason adenocarcinoma is the commonest endometrial carcinoma.

The cervical canal is lined internally with secretory columnar epithelium, whilst the vaginal portion is covered by squamous epithelium.

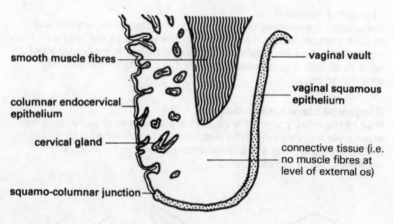

smooth muscle fibres

vaginal vault

vaginal squamous epithelium

columnar endocervical epithelium

cervical gland

connective tissue (i.e. no muscle fibres at level of external os)

squamo-columnar junction

Fig. 8 Histology of the uterine cervix

'Migration' of the squamo-columnar junction outwards results in the columnar epithelium becoming visible on speculum examination: the so-called cervical erosion (common before the age of 20, in pregnancy, and in women on the pill).

Carcinoma-in-situ of the cervix normally arises in the transition zone where epithelium is undergoing squamous metaplasia. Carcinoma-in-situ (CIN 3: cervical intra-epithelial neoplasia 3) may go on to develop a squamous cell carcinoma of the cervix, in one woman in *six*, over a period of about 6 years.

2. THE OVARY

Size, shape and position

The ovary is an almond shaped organ approximately 1 1/2" (3.8 cm) long in the reproductive years, attached to the back of the broad ligament by the mesovarium. It is attached to the uterus by the round ligament of the ovary, which represents the remains of the upper half of the gubernaculum.

Blood supply and lymphatics

Blood supply: The ovary is supplied by the ovarian artery which (for embryological reasons) arises from the aorta at the level of the renal arteries.

Lymphatics: Mainly to the para-aortic nodes, along the course of the ovarian arteries, but also to the uterine fundus, and so to the contralateral ovary.

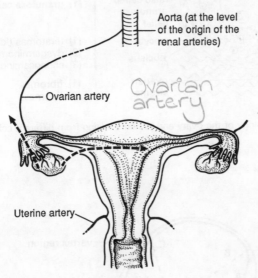

Aorta (at the level of the origin of the renal arteries)

Ovarian artery

Uterine artery

Fig. 9 Lymphatic drainage of the ovaries: drainage follows the direction of the dotted lines

Histology

The histology of the ovary provides one of the few ways of rationalising neoplastic tumours by cell of origin (see Fig. 10).

3. FETAL ANATOMY

Although the fetal shoulders represent its widest part (bisacromial diameter), they seldom cause problems in labour and in practice it is the presenting part, usually the fetal head, that matters. The various parts and diameters are shown in Figure 11.

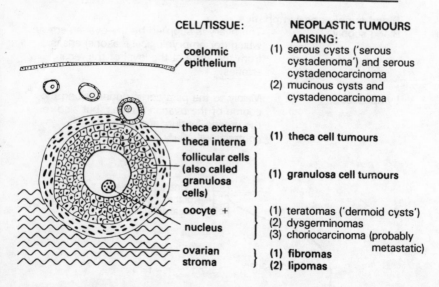

CELL/TISSUE:	NEOPLASTIC TUMOURS ARISING:
coelomic epithelium	(1) serous cysts ('serous cystadenoma') and serous cystadenocarcinoma
	(2) mucinous cysts and cystadenocarcinoma
theca externa theca interna	(1) theca cell tumours
follicular cells (also called granulosa cells)	(1) granulosa cell tumours
oocyte + nucleus	(1) teratomas ('dermoid cysts') (2) dysgerminomas (3) choriocarcinoma (probably metastatic)
ovarian stroma	(1) fibromas (2) lipomas

Fig. 10 Histology of the ovary and tumours arising from different cell types

fetal head diameters

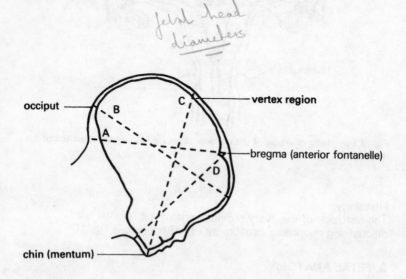

occiput

B

C — vertex region

A

bregma (anterior fontanelle)

D

chin (mentum)

Fig. 11 Parts of the fetal head and the important diameters of the fetal head; for explanation of diameters A–D see Table 2

Table 2. Fetal head diameters (*measurements in cm*)

Diameter	Presentation	Name of diameter	Average size (cm)
A	Vertex	Suboccipito-bregmatic	10
B	Poorly flexed vertex	Occipito-frontal	12
C	Brow	Mento-vertical	13
D	Face	Submento-bregmatic	10

Note that the degree of flexion of the fetal head in relation to the fetal neck will define its presentation, and so the presenting diameter. The normal presentation is by the vertex, the neck being well flexed.

The fetal head is said to be engaged when its greatest diameter (bi-parietal diameter) has passed through the pelvic inlet. Since this is assumed to be the smallest pelvic diameter, it is implied that once the head is engaged, labour will not become obstructed.

4. PLACENTAL ANATOMY

The placenta is a disc of tissue made up of approximately 20 cotyledons. The cord normally enters it roughly in the centre. Various placental anomalies exist including:

Battledore placenta: Cord enters the placenta at the side (marginal insertion).

Velamentous insertion: The umbilicial vessels run in the membranes before entering the placenta. (May cause vasa praevia.)

Bipartite placenta: The placenta is divided into two separate lobes, joined by vessels running in the membranes.

Succenturate placenta: An accessory separate cotyledon is joined to the main placenta by vessels running in the membranes. (May cause vasa praevia.)

These anomalies may result in:

- accidental damage to the umbilical vessels at the time of membrane rupture
- accidental retention of products of conception when the placenta consists of two or more parts.

5. PHYSIOLOGY

The menstrual cycle

Understanding the menstrual cycle is essential to the understanding of gynaecological endocrinology. The events that make up the cycle are as follows:

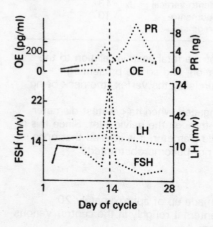

(a) Early follicular phase: low oestrogen and progesterone levels cause positive feedback stimulation secretion of FSH (and LH), levels of which therefore rise: the increased FSH level stimulates follicular development (but note FSH does not *initiate* follicular development).

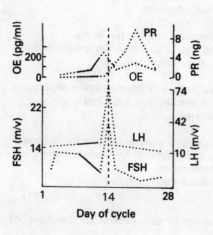

(b) Late follicular phase: as the developing follicle matures, it secretes increasing amounts of oestrogen, which at the initially lower concentrations causes negative feedback inhibition of FSH, levels of which therefore fall.

Fig. 12 The menstrual cycle: OE = oestrogen; PR = progesterone; FSH = follicle stimulating hormone; LH = luteinizing hormone; O = LH surge: ovulation occurs approximately 12 hours later

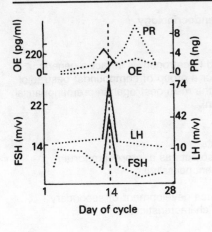

(c) LH surge and ovulation: at higher levels, oestrogen causes positive feedback stimulation of LH secretion, resulting in the LH surge, and, 12 hours later, ovulation.

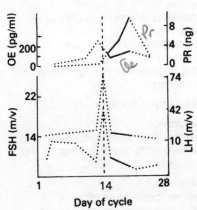

(d) Early luteal phase: oestrogen levels decrease initially, probably due to follicular disruption; the corpus luteum then starts to secrete increasing amounts of progesterone (and some oestrogen) and FSH and LH levels drop, due to negative feedback inhibition, so preventing any further follicular development.

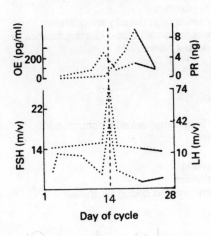

(e) Late luteal phase: in the event of no pregnancy, the corpus luteum fails and progesterone levels drop, so removing the negative feedback inhibition of FSH (and LH), levels of which therefore start to rise, so stimulating the further development of a new follicle.

Obstetric and gynaecological endocrinology

Oestrogen

Chemical nature: Steroid ('oestrogen' is in fact a generic term for a group of compounds: oestradiol being the main oestrogen in premenopausal women).

Produced by: Ovary
Placenta
Fat (also acts as a 'store' [important postmenopausally]).

Actions: Promotes development of secondary sexual characteristics.

Menstruation:
  endometrial proliferation (proliferative phase)
  promotes secretory phase (with progesterone)
  provides feedback to the hypothalamus and pituitary.

Stimulates oocyte development.

During pregnancy:
  stimulates breast development
  stimulates myometrial hypertrophy and hyperplasia.

Metabolic effects:
  encourages calcification of bone
  increases circulating cholesterol and triglycerides
  decreases high density lipoproteins
  increases certain blood clotting factors
  decreases fibrinolysis.

Progesterone

Chemical nature: Steroid.

Produced by: Ovary (with small adrenal contribution).
Placenta.

Actions: (requires oestrogen to work)
  Causes changes in vaginal epithelium
  Cervical mucus decreases in amount and becomes thicker

Promotes secretory changes in endometrium
Raises uterine excitation threshold, so relaxing uterine muscle
    during pregnancy
Generalised smooth muscle relaxation
Stimulates glandular development in breast
Metabolic effects — generally catabolic.

Human placental lactogen

Chemical nature: Protein (similar to growth hormone and prolactin).

Secreted by: The placenta. Level rises during pregnancy and then plateaus at 35 weeks.

Actions: ? Alters carbohydrate metabolism (anti-insulin—growth-hormone- like effect). Pregnancy can apparently progress normally without it.

Human chorionic gonadotrophin

Chemical nature: Protein (similar to pituitary LH).

Secreted by: The placenta. Level peaks at 12 weeks and then falls off.

Actions: Early — prolongs corpus luteum
Late — ? controls progesterone metabolism.

Follicle stimulating hormone (FSH)

Chemical nature: Glycoprotein.

Secreted by: Pituitary under control of GnRH (q.v.).

Actions: Stimulates follicular growth (but does not initiate it).

Luteinising hormone (LH)

Chemical nature: Glycoprotein.

Secreted by: Pituitary under control of GnRH (q.v.).

Actions: Stimulates ovulation
Follicular steroidogenesis
Follicular maturation and rupture
Luteinises the corpus luteum.

Prolactin

Chemical nature:	Polypeptide.
Secreted by:	Pituitary.
Actions:	Initially stimulates milk secretion High levels inhibit ovarian oestrogen secretion.

Gonadotrophin releasing hormone (GnRH)

Chemical nature:	Decapeptide.
Secreted by:	The hypothalamus.
Actions:	Stimulates FSH and LH secretion.

Landmarks in fetal development

2–3 days post-conception:	Implantation.
3–4 weeks post-conception:	Heart starts to beat (detectable by ultrasound scan from 6 weeks' *gestation*).
8 weeks:	Majority of organ development has occurred and further development is by growth.
16–18 weeks (multigravidas)	
18–20 weeks (primigravidas):	Quickening (mother first notices fetal movements).
24 weeks:	Fetus viable. Stillbirth registerable.
Approximately 26 weeks:	Fetal heart beat first detectable clinically (i.e. by fetal stethoscope).
32 weeks:	Fetal outcome as good as at term in special centres.
34 weeks:	Surfactant production starts to rise.
38 weeks + :	Term (i.e. delivery at this time carries minimum perinatal risk).
40 weeks + :	*Post term.*

Gynaecology

Gynaecological symptomatology

GYNAECOLOGICAL SYMPTOMATOLOGY

Menstrual disturbances — see p. 30 Urological disorders — see p. 75.

Both in clinical practice and in examinations the question frequently arises as to what pathology may be responsible for particular symptoms. Usually this information can only be presented in bare list form, but below an attempt is made to present these lists in the most rational manner, a system which it is hoped may aid recall.

As a general rule it is better to learn broad headings before specific causes, partly because this provides a rational route of recall, and partly because it avoids concentrating on obscure and unimportant causes of a certain condition.

Figure 13 provides a guide to the clerking of gynaecological patients. Fertility patients are clerked on a separate questionnaire required for the investigation of those patients. These questionnaires can be obtained from Mr. Webb's secretary.

DYSPAREUNIA

Definition: Painful and/or difficult sexual intercourse.

Classifications: Onset:
          Primary — always been present
          Secondary — acquired after previous
             pain-free intercourse.
       Anatomical:
          Superficial — felt at or around introitus
          Deep — felt deep in pelvis.

Superficial dyspareunia
Most commonly due to thrush. Post-episiotomy discomfort is also common and almost always settles without revision of the scar.

GYNAECOLOGICAL QUESTIONNAIRE FOR MEDICAL STUDENTS

Age; Race; Occupation

Date of last normal menstrual period

Parity + miscarriages + terminations of pregnancy. Were the babies delivered normally?

When was the last cervical smear taken? Was it normal? Has the patient ever had an abnormal smear?

History of Present Complaint

Emphasise the important points in this part of the history.
Don't get bogged down in detail.
Ask **relevant** direct questions.
Abdomino-pelvic pain should lead to questions about bowel habit, the presence or absence of blood or slime in the motions, indigestion and vomiting, dysuria and haematuria.

Gynaecological History

Age at Menarche   Cycle: length of flow/length of cycle
                                                 heavy or light
                                                 painful or not

IMB?   PCB?   Dyspareunia?

Abnormal vaginal discharge?

Contraception?

PH of STD?

Age of patient's mother's menopause?

Control of micturition: does she suffer from stress or urgency incontinence?

If menopausal, age at menopause, and has there been any PMB?

Past Medical History

As usual.

Family History

Have any female relatives suffered from ovarian cancer?

Any DM, thyroid problems, hypertension etc.

Social History

Smokes?   Alcohol?

Drug history   Allergies?

If the patient does not have an occupation, determine the partner's job and, if relevant, enquire into the social circumstances.

Fig. 13 Gynaecological questionnaire providing a guide to the clerking of gynaecological patients

Causes: Psychological/vaginismus (= spasm of
levator ani):
postnatal depression
fear of further pregnancies
perception that delivery was very
unpleasant
Vaginal dryness whilst breast feeding or
due to progestogen-only pill
Infections/inflammation of the vulva and
vagina:
Candida
Trichomonas vaginalis
Bartholin's cyst/abscess
atrophic vaginitis
vulval dystrophies
Local lesions causing vaginal narrowing:
post-episiotomy scarring
vaginal repair surgery
Rare congenital abnormalities, e.g. vaginal
septum, absent vagina
Imperforate hymen.

Deep dyspareunia

Causes: Pelvic inflammatory disease — acute and
chronic (including cervicitis)
Endometriosis
Pelvic tumours
Ectopic pregnancy
Loaded sigmoid colon
Spastic colon/irritable bowel syndrome
Possibly retroverted uterus and/or
prolapsed ovaries (opinions vary) — so-
called 'collision dyspareunia'.
Psychosexual disorders should not be
forgotten: psychiatric opinion prior to
surgery may be wise.

MENORRHAGIA/MENSTRUAL DISORDERS — SEE P. 30

DYSMENORRHOEA

Definition: Painful menstruation (sufficient to be
socially inconvenient and adversely affect
the quality of the woman's life, as most
women have some degree of discomfort
associated with their periods).

Classification:

Primary dysmenorrhoea (idiopathic, intrinsic, spasmodic dysmenorrhoea):
Patient is usually nulliparous
Pain starts with flow of menses, and disappears within 1–2 days
Low crampy midline pain, often associated with autonomic nervous system disturbance — nausea, vomiting and diarrhoea
Probably due to release of prostaglandins into circulation at time of menstruation
Not associated with other gynaecological pathology.

Secondary dysmenorrhoea (acquired, extrinsic, congestive dysmenorrhoea):
Pain begins up to 5 days premenstrually and reaches a peak either with commencement of menstruation or with peak of flow, settling soon afterwards
Constant (as opposed to crampy) pain, often lateralised to one side
Patient is usually over 20 years old
Usually associated with and secondary to organic pelvic pathology, e.g. endometriosis, pelvic inflammatory disease.

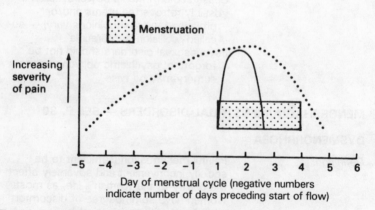

Fig. 14 Relationship of pain to menstrual flow in primary dysmenorrhoea (solid line) and secondary dysmenorrhoea (dotted line)

PELVIC PAIN

Acute pelvic pain

Causes:

All the causes of chronic pelvic pain (q.i.)
Associated with pregnancy:
  ectopic pregnancy
  abortion
Complications of ovarian cysts, e.g.
  torsion, haemorrhage, corpus luteum
  rupture
Dysmenorrhoea (q.v.)
Infections and inflammations (especially
  chlamydia and gonorrhoea) — 'pelvic
  inflammatory disease'
Complications of fibroids, e.g. red
  degeneration of pregnancy
Uterine contractions in trying to expel
  items from uterine cavity, e.g. polyp,
  intra-uterine contraceptive device
Mittelschmerz
Non-gynaecological causes of acute
  pelvic/lower abdominal pain, e.g.
  appendicitis, diverticulitis, cystitis
Irritable bowel syndrome
Psychological problems, e.g. past history
  of sexual abuse as a child.

Chronic Pelvic Pain

Causes:

Infections — 'chronic pelvic inflammatory
  disease'
Endometriosis
Pelvic tumours, malignant and non-
  malignant, gynaecological and colonic
Non-gynaecological causes of chronic
  pelvic/lower abdominal pain:
  constipation/bowel disease (including
  irritable bowel syndrome)
  orthopaedic disease (especially
  referred pain from spine)
  urological disease.

Pelvic malignancy can cause pain felt in the leg and hip and mimic
lumbo-sacral spinal disorders.

PRURITUS VULVAE

90% of cases in practice are thrush. Always exclude diabetes.

Definition:	Itching of the vulva, generally taken to include the perineal and peri-anal skin. .
Causes:	Irritation secondary to vaginal discharge (q.v.)
	Vulval infections — bacterial, fungal, viral (NB herpes genitalis is usually painful)
	Vulval infestations, e.g. lice, scabies
	Bartholin's cyst — usually painless
	Bartholin's abscess — very painful
	Neoplasms — vulval, vaginal (often symptomless unless they bleed)
	Vulval dystrophies, atrophic and hypertrophic
	Urological disease, e.g. incontinence
	Dermatological disorders which happen to affect the vulva
	Systemic disease causing general or local pruritus, e.g. diabetes mellitus (± associated fungal infection), liver disease, uraemia
	Local (anal) disease, e.g. piles
	Psychosomatic/stress related.

VAGINAL DISCHARGE

Classification	Normal — non irritant and non-offensive, clear mucoid discharge; heavier mid-cycle at ovulation; contains vaginal skin cells and may cause beige stain on underclothes
	Cervicitis — milky viscoid
	Vaginal infections:
	candida — white, curdlike
	Trichomonas vaginalis — frothy, yellow-green
	Pyogenic — foul-smelling, brown, watery
	Neoplasms, e.g. uterine, cervical, vaginal —foul-smelling, brown, water (often associated with infection)
	Foreign bodies (common cause of discharge in pre-pubertal age group), including tampons
	Fistulae — urinary and faecal
	Miscellaneous (non-pathological) — semen, douches, pessaries.

GALACTORRHOEA

Definition:	Inappropriate, non-puerperal lactation.
Causes:	Prolactin-secreting pituitary tumours Drugs, e.g. phenothiazines, oral contraceptive pill, methyldopa Ectopic prolactin secretion, e.g. bronchogenic carcinoma Hypothalamic lesion/pituitary stalk section Hypothyroidism.

MITTELSCHMERZ

Definition:	Cyclical intermenstrual pain associated with ovulation.
Features:	Common: up to 25% of women experience mid-cycle discomfort Ovarian in origin Ranges from mild discomfort to severe pain Usually a non-cramping, non-radiation, short-lasting pain, occurring only at mid-cycle which may or may not be associated with ovulation bleeding ('spotting') May alternate from right to left side in different cycles (often helpful diagnostically) Combined oral contraceptive pill 'cures' it.

HIRSUTISM

Definition:	Excess growth of hair in abnormal place on the body, i.e. non-female pattern hair on a female.
Pathophysiological mechanisms:	Physiological/racial, e.g. southern European and Asian women Increased circulating androgens Increased end organ response.

Causes: Physiological — racial and familial variation,
              pregnancy and post menopausally
              Iatrogenic — drugs, e.g. phenytoin,
              steroids, anti-gonadotrophins
              Genetic abnormalities, e.g. intersex
              Endocrine disorders:
                  adrenal/ovarian: polycystic ovarian
                                  syndrome
                                  adrenal hyperplasia
                                  masculinising ovarian
                                      tumours
                                  adrenal cortex
                                      tumours
                                  Cushing's syndrome
              Others, e.g.   acromegaly

VIRILISM

This is a more generalised effect involving the development of male
secondary sexual characteristics including:
    clitoral hypertrophy
    breast atrophy
    male pattern. baldness
    deepening of the voice
    excessive body hair, i.e. hirsutism.

ACUTE VAGINAL BLEEDING

This is a common presenting symptom of gynaecological and
obstetrical disorder in the Casualty Department. The condition may
be life-threatening and urgent resuscitation with uncrossmatched
blood may be required.

Causes: Ectopic pregnancy
              Abortion — especially incomplete abortion
              Intra-uterine contraceptive device (usually
                  recently fitted)
              Heavy menstrual flow
              Ovulation — 'mid-cycle spotting'
              Post-coital bleeding (q.v.)
              Obstetric causes — show, abruption,
                  placenta praevia
              Vaginal laceration.

SEXUAL DYSFUNCTION (WOMEN AND MEN)

Table 3. Classification of sexual dysfunction in women and men

Aspect of sexuality affected	Sexual dysfunction	
	Women	Men
Sexual interest	Impaired	Impaired
Arousal	Impaired	Erectile dysfunction
Orgasm	Orgasmic dysfunction	Premature ejaculation
		Retarded ejaculation Ejaculatory pain
Other types of dysfunction	Vaginismus Dyspareunia Sexual phobias	Dyspareunia Sexual phobias

Psychological causes of sexual dysfunction

Predisposing factors: Restrictive upbringing
Disturbed family relations
Inadequate sexual information
Traumatic early sexual experiences
Child sexual abuse.

Precipitants: Childbirth
Discord in general relationship
Infidelity
Unreasonable expectations
Partner dysfunctions
Random failure
Reaction to organic factors
Ageing
Anxiety/depression
Traumatic sexual experiences.

Maintaining factors: Performance anxiety
Anticipation of failure
Guilt
Loss of attraction between partners
Poor communication between partners
Fear of intimacy
Impaired self-image
Restricted foreplay
Psychiatric disorder.

Abnormal menstrual and non-menstrual genital bleeding

Abnormal menstrual and non-menstrual genital bleeding are frequent and important gynaecological symptoms, with a significance ranging from crippling heavy periods unassociated with serious underlying pathology, to the scant spotting which may be the only clue to an endometrial carcinoma. The main headings under which abnormal genital bleeding is considered are:

- Abnormal menstrual bleeding
- Non-menstrual bleeding
  — associated with pregnancy
  — not associated with pregnancy.

Definitions:

Menarche:	Age of onset of menstruation. Normal range in UK 10–16 years; average age 13 1/2 years.
Menopause:	Age at cessation of menstruation. Normal range in UK 45–60 years; average age 51 years (see p. 87).
Climacteric:	The period (as opposed to specific age) during which a woman changes from reproductive to non-reproductive ability, characterised by hot flushes and sweats.
Dysfunctional uterine bleeding:	Abnormal uterine bleeding for which no organic cause can be found. The abnormality is assumed to be a disorder of the hypothalamic/pituitary/ovarian axis.

ABNORMAL MENSTRUAL BLEEDING

The terminology surrounding abnormal menstrual bleeding is confusing, many terms meaning different things to different people.

For this reason the authors prefer the use of plain English (thus 'D & C for menorrhagia' becomes less ambiguous as 'D & C for heavy periods'). None the less, the formal terms are encountered and should be understood, and are therefore included below.

In general terms it will be noted that abnormalities of flow are usually due to local/genital causes, whilst abnormalities of cycle timing are often due to systemic/endocrine causes.

NB Psycho-social problems may present as menstrual abnormality.

Menorrhagia

Definition: Cyclical menstrual bleeding which is excessive in amount. No abnormality of cycle is implied, but one may be present.

Features: Presents with excessive use of towels/tampons; passing clots, flooding and/or anaemia.

Causes: Uterine polyps
Uterine fibroids
Endometrial hyperplasia (q.v.)
Pelvic inflammatory disease
Adenomyosis
Endocrine disturbances:
          hypothyroidism
          anovular cycles
Systemic disease, e.g. liver disease
Dysfunctional uterine bleeding
Bleeding diathesis — should be excluded in
          the young teenager.

Cryptomenorrhoea (hypomenorrhoea)

Definition: Cyclical menstrual bleeding of abnormally small quantity (or spotting which may occur at any time). No abnormality of cycle is implied, but one may be present.

Features: Minimal menstrual loss, which may only amount to a smear on the underwear.

Causes: Endocrine disorders, e.g.:
          hyperthyroidism
          hyperprolactinaemia
          polycystic ovarian syndrome

Scarring and obliteration of the
endometrial cavity: (Asherman's
syndrome)
General debility, e.g. tuberculosis
'Physiological', i.e. as a normal variant
Oral contraceptive use
Life event/stress:
  change of job
  moving house
  weight loss/anorexia nervosa.

Polymenorrhoea

Definition: Abnormally frequent (21 days) menstrual
cycle. No abnormality of flow is implied,
but one may be present.

Features: Self-evident condition, usually associated
with anovulatory cycles.

Causes: Corpus luteum insufficiency
Ovulatory failure
Disturbance of the
  hypothalamic/pituitary/ovarian axis.

Oligomenorrhoea

Definition: Infrequent menstruation occurring at
intervals in between 6 weeks and 6
months. The causes are those of
amenorrhoea (q.v.).

Amenorrhoea

Definition: Absence of menstruation for 6 months or
more. See p. 84.

Metrorrhagia

Definition: Irregular vaginal bleeding occuring in
between apparently normal periods.
Synonymous with intermenstrual bleeding
(q.v.).

Metropathia haemorrhagica

Definition: Excessive menses at long intervals
associated histologically with cystic
endometrial hyperplasia, usually associated
with anovulatory cycles.

MANAGEMENT OF ABNORMAL MENSTRUAL BLEEDING

Adequate history and examination (general and pelvic).

Investigations:	Full blood count (for anaemia)
	Biochemistry (e.g. LFT's)
	21-day progesterone (if infertility is an associated problem)
	Endocrine investigation (e.g. thyroid function tests)
	Serum iron studies.

as clinically indicated

D & C: opinions vary concerning the timing (and indeed the necessity in some patients) of this procedure. A standard plan would be:

- age 20 or less and adequate responses to hormone treatment (q.v.) — D & C not necessary
- age 20–40 and no suspicion of organic disease — D & C required, but may be deferred
- age over 40 — D & C essential.

Hysteroscopy increases accuracy of diagnosis and enables directed therapy, e.g. polypectomy.

Other procedures, e.g. laparoscopy, may be needed in obscure cases in which there is suspicion of organic disease.

Treatment: the underlying disease is treated where appropriate. The remainder of patients will be said to have 'dysfunctional uterine bleeding', i.e. of no known cause: for these patients the treatment must be tailored to the severity of the bleeding and the individual patient's needs. Available options include:

- general measures, e.g. correcting anaemia
- hysteroscopy and D & C in themselves may be therapeutic
- polypectomy
- hormone treatment, e.g. OCP, progestogens, danazol, HRT, (treatment of choice in younger patients)
- epsi-aminocaproic acid
- myomectomy
- hysterectomy.

The management of abnormal menstrual bleeding is summarised in the flow chart on page 34.

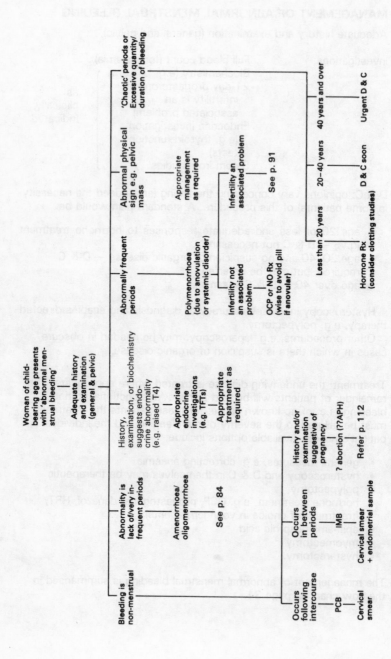

Fig. 15 Abnormal menstrual bleeding

ENDOMETRIAL HYPERPLASIA

Incidence increases in the last menstrual decade. Two types exist, differentiated histologically. Both cause abnormal uterine bleeding:

Cystic hyperplasia

Benign Caused by unopposed oestrogen stimulation Often associated with the clinical picture called 'metropathia haemorrhagica' (q.v.) Histologically recognised by 'Swiss cheese' appearance (large dilated endometrial glands) Responds to progesterone treatment.

Adenomatous (atypical) hyperplasia

20% risk of progression to invasive carcinoma Dependent on but not caused by oestrogen Histologically only endometrial glands are involved (cf. cystic hyperplasia in which there is a more general hyperplasia) Treatment: hysterectomy.

NON-MENSTRUAL BLEEDING

Definition: Any vaginal bleeding not associated with menstruation.
Unlike disordered menstrual bleeding, an identifiable pathological cause can usually be found.

Classification: Intermenstrual bleeding:
      bleeding in between periods
Post-coital bleeding:
      bleeding after sexual intercourse
Post-menopausal bleeding:
      bleeding more than 6 months after cessation of menstruation
Bleeding in pregnancy (q.v.).

Common and/or important causes

Usefully considered anatomically. Those marked * are especially common.

Vulva and vagina: Carcinoma
Inflammations
Urethral caruncle.

Cervix: 'Erosions'
Polyp*
Carcinoma and CIN (cervical intra-epithelial neoplasia).

Uterine body:	Abortion* IUCD* Polyps Hyperplasia Carcinoma Breakthrough bleeding (from OCP) and 'spotting' at time of ovulation HRT.
Ovaries and fallopian tubes:	Fallopian tube carcinoma (rare) Oestrogen-secreting ovarian tumours (by their effect on the endometrium — unopposed by progesterone — causing hyperplasia).

Management:	Because of the risk of carcinoma in non-menstrual bleeding, urgent investigation and appropriate treatment is mandatory in all cases. Usually this takes the form of:
	    examination under anaesthesia
	    hysteroscopy
	    D & C.
	(Endometrial biopsies may be taken in out-patients, with vacuum devices.)

Gynaecological infections and inflammations

Inflammation, (including that due to infection), is a common gynaecological problem, and any part of the genital tract may be involved:

- Vulvitis, including abscess of Bartholin's gland
- Vaginitis, including abscess of Skene's gland
- Cervicitis
- Endometritis and pyometra
- Salpingitis
- Oöphoritis
- Venereal diseases.

Pelvic inflammatory disease is a general term for acute or chronic infection of the tubes and ovaries, often with involvement of the adjacent tissues.

VULVITIS

inflammation of the vulva may be acute or chronic.

Aetiology

Infections:	Fungal infections, especially in the elderly, diabetics and after antibiotic therapy *Trichomonas vaginalis* Venereal diseases Warts Herpes genitalis (Burning vulva syndrome — associated with human papillomavirus).
Infestations:	Pediculosis pubis Threadworms.
Mechanical/chemical:	Trauma Poor hygiene Urinary and faecal contamination Allergy to perfumes, soap, talc, Dettol etc.

Miscellaneous:	Atrophic and dystrophic conditions Carcinoma Skin disorders — eczema, psoriasis, contact dermatitis, etc.

Signs and symptoms

Acute:	Pruritus
	Burning
	Erythema
	Oedema
	Bleeding
	Pain — may be very severe leading to an
	   inability to walk or sit, and acute
	   retention of urine
	Ulceration and/or vesicles.

Chronic:	Less severe inflammation with minimal
	   oedema
	Severe pruritus → excoriation → secondary
	   infection
	Area involved may include:
	   mons
	   perineum
	   anus
	   anal canal
	   adjacent thighs
	Ulcerative lesions may be due to:
	   granuloma
	   carcinoma
	   melanoma
	End result may be destruction of the vulva.

Diagnosis

History
General physical examination
Cervical and vulvar cytology
Local, endocervical, vaginal, urethral and anal canal swabs
Full blood count and ESR
Urinalysis
Appropriate test for venereal disease if suspected.

Treatment

General treatments:	Sitz baths
	Good local hygiene
	Avoid:
	   soaps
	   perfumes

talcs
sprays
bath-oils
nylon underwear, tights and
trousers
Dry area thoroughly with hair-dryer after
washing
Oral antihistamines (which also cause
sedation which may reduce excoriation),
but avoid local antihistamines and local
anaesthetics which can themselves
cause sensitivity reactions
Topical steroids (*only* after treating local
infective causes)
Treating local irritation and cause will
reduce trauma/excoriation.

Specific treatments: Education of elderly patients who may well
apply Dettol to the vulva to treat an
'infection' which commonly results in a
chemical vulvitis.

Lice: Gamma-benzene hexachloride.

Scabies: Benzyl benzoate; malathion

Threadworms: Cause pruritus mainly at night: eradicate
with piperazine citrate.

Candidiasis: Treat diabetes mellitus if present
Topical antifungals
Topical antifungals + steroid
Treat vaginal moniliasis.

Trichomonas vaginalis: Metronidazole 400 mg three times a day
for 10 days
Avoid intercourse for 2 weeks.
(It is only necessary to treat a woman's
consort if intercourse is not avoided for
this length of time.)

Warts: Local treatment with:
podophyllin
silver nitrate
cautery (diathermy)
excision
freezing
laser
Treat the partner.

VENEREAL DISEASES

Syphilis
Gonorrhoea
Chancroid
Non-specific urethritis
Herpes genitalis
Lymphogranuloma venereum
Granuloma inguinale
Trichomonas vaginalis
HIV.

Syphilis

Syphilis is caused by the spirochaete *Treponema pallidum*. It may be congenital (i.e. contracted in utero), or acquired; the former may result in abortion, fetal death, or congenital abnormality. In adults and children the disease may be active and florid, or latent. Any tissue of the body may be affected.

Stages

Primary (very infectious):
3–6 weeks after infection through an abrasion, a chancre forms. Spirochaetes can be obtained and identified under dark-ground illumination. Rarely observed in women. Often on the cervix but also on the vulva, lip, finger, anus
Almost painless
Rubbery, painless glands
Spontaneous healing with slight scar.

Secondary (moderately infectious):
2 months after chancre
Varied dermatological lesions which can mimic any lesion. Often a coppery coloured, maculo-papular rash
80% have muco-cutaneous lesion
50% have generalised lymphadenopathy
Alopecia
Condylomata lata
Rash heals with no scar, but may leave depigmentation or hyperpigmentation.

Tertiary (rarely infectious):
Appears within 3–10 years
Gumma, due to endarteritis, of:
skin
bone
viscera.

| | Cardiovascular syphilis:
    aortitis
    aneurysms
Periostitis
Neurosyphilis:
    tabes dorsalis
    charcot's joints
    general paralysis of the insane. |

Diagnosis: Positive Romberg's sign   ⎫
                      Absent joint position   ⎬ neurosyphilis.
                        sensation   ⎭
                      Argyll Robertson pupils

Serology: VDRL (screening test; +ve after 5–6
                      weeks, but don't forget yaws)
                  FTA-ABS (most sensitive; +ve 3–4
                      weeks)
                  RPCFT
                  TPHA
                  TPI.

Dark-ground illumination.

Treatment: Penicillin 600,000 u/day i.m. daily for 10
                  days *or* 2.4 million u i.m. stat.
                  Contact tracing
                  (Erythromycin 500 mg four times a day
                      for 15 days in those allergic to
                      penicillin).

NB Remember the Herxheimer reaction.

Gonorrhoea

Gonorrhoea is a common infection caused by *Neisseria gonorrhoeae*, a Gram-negative, kidney-shaped, paired, usually intracellular organism. Symptoms usually appear 1–3 weeks after infection although up to 60% of women may be asymptomatic. *Trichomonas vaginalis* infection in the same patient is common. The adult vaginal epithelium is resistant to the organism which therefore colonises the:

- cervix
- urethra
- Skene's gland
- Bartholin's gland
- anus.

Subsequent ascending infection to the endometrium, tubes and ovaries is common, with the formation of tubo-ovarian abscesses, and subsequent infertility.

Clinical manifestations of infection:
Dysuria
Discharge
Abscess: Urethral
                                 Cervical
                                 Skene's gland
                                 Bartholin's gland
                                 Tubo-ovarian
Vulvitis
Vaginitis (in children)
Dissemination via
    bloodstream causing: Iritis
                           Arthritis
                           Endo–carditis
Opthalmia neonatorum
    in neonates.

Diagnosis: Gram-stained smear
                                 Culture (difficult)
                                 GCFT (becomes positive after 6 weeks)
                                 Reliable serology not available.

Treatment: Penicillin (if not resistant) 4.8 mega-units
                                     i.m. after probenecid 1 g orally 1/2 hour
                                     before
                                 NB *Always* obtain blood for syphilis
                                     serology before starting treatment.
OR   Ampicillin 3.5 g orally after probenecid
OR   Tetracycline 1.5 g stat. orally, then 0.5 g
                                     few times a day for 4 days.

1 week after treatment check that the patient is not infectious. Check again at 2 weeks. Re-treat as required.

NB Be aware of more modern antibiotics becoming available and check, *before* your final examinations, the latest treatment regimes in your hospital's Department of Genitourinary Medicine.

Chancroid
Chancroid is an acute, contagious, localised lesion, consisting of small, painful, shallow irregular ulcers, associated with suppurating inguinal lymph nodes. It is caused by the short, slender, Gram-negative bacillus, *Haemophilus ducreyi*.

Diagnosis:	Clinical findings.
Treatment:	Sulphonamides (sulphadimidine 4 g daily for 10–14 days) Aspirate bubos (do not incise) Review patient for 3 months.

Non-specific urethritis (NSU)

The development of more accurate diagnostic techniques has reduced the number of infections ascribed to non-specific genital infection.

Organisms:	*Chlamydia trachomatis* *Mycoplasma hominis* — T strains.
Features:	Usually no symptoms, but may cause: vaginal discharge mild dysuria frequency pelvic pain subsequent tubal infertility dyspareunia Reiter's syndrome Fitzhugh–Curtis syndrome — pelvic pain plus pain around liver.

Symptomatic in males who may develop Reiter's syndrome, a serious complication, features of which are:

conjunctivitis
uveitis
polyarthritis.

Diagnosis:	By excluding: gonorrhoea trichomonas candidiasis other causes of discharge.
Treatment:	Always treat the female partner of an affected male Oxytetracycline 1 g daily for 2–3 weeks Erythromycin stearate 1 g daily for 2–3 weeks Tarivid (ofloxacin) 2 tablets daily for 5–10 days No intercourse or alcohol 20% relapse rate (reduced using ofloxacin).

Herpes genitalis

Herpes genitalis is the commonest cause of ulceration of the vulva and cervix. It is caused by herpes hominis virus type 2, and is moderately contagious, developing 4–7 days after intercourse. Relapses occur due to the carrier state.

Features:	Itching and soreness before vesicles
	Severe pain with primary infection requiring opioids
	Secondary infection can occur
	Acute retention of urine requires catheterisation
	Sacral radiculitis may occur
	Clinical diagnosis confirmed by virus culture.
Treatment:	Symptomatic
	Idoxuridine
	Acyclovir
	No known cure.

Lymphogranuloma venereum

This is a contagious infection caused by a chlamydial organism.

Features:	Transient primary lesion
	Suppurative lymphangitis
	Serious local complications:
	oedema
	ulcer
	fistula.
Diagnosis:	Frei intra-dermal test.
Treatment:	Tetracycline 500 mg 6 hourly orally for 14 days
	Ofloxacin
	Aspirate bubos
	Follow-up patient for 6 months.

Granuloma inguinale

This is a chronic granulomatous condition of the genitals which is rare in temperate climates, caused by a Gram-negative rod-shaped bacillus, *Donovania granulomatis*.

Features:	No lymphadenopathy
	Granulomatous mass
	Slow healing and scarring.

Diagnosis:	Donovan bodies.
Treatment:	Streptomycin or tetracyclines.

Trichomonas vaginalis

Trichomonas vaginalis, a flagellate *protozoan* 15–30 μm long, with four flagellae and a membrane, is a common cause of infection in young women (up to 20%).

Clinical features:	Vaginitis Urethritis Cystitis Copious green/yellow offensive frothy discharge Irritation Soreness Dyspareunia Dysuria Symptom-free carriers Frequently associated with gonorrhoea.
Diagnosis:	Direct microscopy Culture Papanicolou smear.

Treatment:	Metronidazole 400 mg three times a day
	    for 10 days
	Avoid intercourse for 14 days (see above)
	Should treat partner at same time although
	    it is reported that organisms in male will
	    die if intercourse avoided for 10 days.

Bartholinitis

Inflammation of Bartholin's gland.

Organisms:	Staphylococci Streptococci *Esch. coli* Gonococcus (rare).

An abscess may develop from an infected cyst.

Treatment:	Incise Drain Marsupialise Culture pus for antibiotic sensitivity.

Marsupialisation, in which the lining of the cavity is sutured to the skin, is a procedure more suited to cysts than abscesses, because in the latter the abscess wall is friable and the tissues oedematous.

Genital warts (syn. condylomata acuminata)
Genital warts are caused by a papillomavirus with an incubation period of 1–6 months. The infection is acquired venereally.

Diagnosis:	Identified by appearance (but must be differentiated from the flat-topped condylomata lata of syphilis) Biopsy (to exclude carcinoma-in-situ and frank carcinoma).
Treatment:	Podophyllin (not in pregnancy) Silver nitrate Cautery Excision Laser.

VAGINITIS AND VAGINAL DISCHARGE

Vaginitis and vaginal discharge can be considered as occurring during three stages of life:

Pre-menarchal

Causes:	Poor hygiene Foreign body (organic or inorganic) Threadworms Sexual interference Sarcoma botyroides (rare cause of bloodstained discharge).
Treatment:	Treat infection agent Remove foreign body (usually during examination under anaesthesia) Local or oral oestrogens are occasionally indicated to mature the vaginal epithelium and thereby increase resistance to infection.

Reproductive period
Heavy 'normal' discharge (usually increased at mid-cycle, due to ovulation, and pre-menstrually). Being pregnant and being on the 'pill' also cause heavy normal discharge.

Specific causes:	*Trichomonas vaginalis* Venereal diseases Streptococci Anaerobic organisms Chlamydia

Retained tampon
Candidiasis (see below)
Non-specific.

Candida albicans (Monilia)
This is a fungus infection, susceptibility to which is increased by oral contraceptives, antibiotics, pregnancy and diabetes mellitus.

Features: Intense irritation and soreness
May spread to the thighs
Thick cheesy discharge
Red inflamed vaginal wall.

Diagnosis: Direct microscopy or Gram-staining (Test urine for sugar).

Treatment: Anti-fungal pessaries and cream
Treat partner if required
Nystatin
Clotrimazole
Miconazole
Oral nystatin eliminates bowel reservoir of fungus.

Non-specific
Sensitivity to contraceptive rubber
Sensitivity to spermicidal creams/foams
Inappropriate chemicals for douching.

Peri/post-menopausal
In the peri– and postmenopausal period, atrophic vaginitis (due to low oestrogen levels) is very common. No specific organism is involved. The patient may complain of prolapse even though none is present.

Features: Purulent often bloodstained discharge
(NB always exclude intra-uterine pathology whenever PMB presents)
Soreness.

Treatment: Local or systemic oestrogens (after excluding malignancy) may be given.

Abscess of Skene's gland
Gland opens at urethral margin
Develops a cyst or abscess.

Differential diagnosis: Urethral diverticulum
Cyst of Gartner's duct (no urethral
connection)
Urethrocoele (mid-line deformity).

TOXIC SHOCK SYNDROME

Definition: A syndrome characterised by:
sudden onset
high fever
vomiting
diarrhoea
confusion
skin rash
predominantly in young women
associated with menses and tampons
infection with *Staph. aureus*
phage group I:
found in vagina in every case
toxic shock toxin = exotoxin
made by above staphylococci
May rapidly progress to severe and
intractable shock.

By 1981 in USA, after publicity and withdrawal of certain tampons,
the incidence dropped sharply.

Treatment: Hospitalise
Intensive care
Remove tampon
Fluid and electrolyte replacement
Blood culture and swabs from mucosal
surfaces
Give β-lactamase-resistant pencillin or
cephalosporin.

CERVICITIS

Inflammation of the cervix which may be acute or chronic. May
spread to uterus and parametrium.

Features: Purulent offensive discharge
May be associated with vulvo-vaginitis
Dyspareunia
Red oedematous cervix
Tender cervix/cervical excitation
Positive laboratory studies for aerobic and
anaerobic pathogens.

Causes:	Acute cervicitis — gonococcus puerperal infection D & C Chronic cervicitis — the sequel of acute cervicitis.
Treatment:	Antibiotics Treat any cervical erosion.

CERVICAL EROSION

Although called an erosion because of its raw appearance, this cervical lesion is not caused by erosion of the ecto-cervical squamous epithelium, but by a down- growth of the endo-cervical columnar epithelium onto the ecto-cervix.

Causes:	Physiological — pregnancy menarche Iatrogenic — combined 'pill' 'mini-pill'.
Features:	Seldom occurs after the menopause May resolve spontaneously (squamous metaplasia → squamous epithelium).

NB Cervical intra-epithelial neoplasia/dysplasia occurs in the transition zone between columnar and squamous epithelium.

Symptoms:	Discharge Intermenstrual bleeding Post-coital bleeding Often asymptomatic.
Treatment (if symptomatic):	Take a cervical smear before: cautery cryocautery laser.

ENDOMETRITIS

This is infection of the endometrium which may occur:

- post-abortion
- postpartum
- post-curettage
- post-IUCD insertion
- postmenopause (atrophic endometritis)

and as a result of:

* ascending gonococcal infection
* descending tuberculous infection (rare).

Features:	Pyrexia Tachycardia Uterine tenderness and dyspareunia Foul lochia Pelvic peritonitis.
Treatment:	Drainage — cervical dilatation Evacuate products of conception if present Antibiotics as appropriate Rest Oestrogens in atrophic cases Supportive therapy Exclude cervical or uterine carcinoma, especially with pyometra.

Salpingitis
Salpingitis is a venereal infection of sexually active women which is commonest in their late teens and early twenties. IUCDs increase the risk, and are therefore not recommended for contraception in young nulliparous women.

Causative organisms:	*Neisseria gonorrhoeae* Chlamydia TB (uncommon).
Pathology:	Ascending vaginal infection ↓ Endocervical glands involved ↓ Superficial endometritis ↓ Endosalpingitis (bilateral) ↓ Exudate, adhesions, tubal occlusion ↓ Tubal abscess ↓ Pelvic peritonitis + oöphoritis Tubo-ovarian abscess Pyosalpinx Hydrosalpinx ↓ Infertility.

Features:	Pain Pyrexia Tenderness + cervical excitation Malaise Dyspareunia Vaginal discharge Urethral discharge and/or — frequency dysuria Dysmenorrhoea Menstrual disorders.
Investigations:	Swabs — urethral endocervical high vaginal rectal (throat) MSU Blood cultures if required.
Treatment:	Antibiotics once specimens taken — a penicillin metronidazole erythromycin or tetracycline or ofloxacin for chlamydia.

Remember to treat the sexual partners if indicated.

OÖPHORITIS/OVARIAN ABSCESS

This is uncommon as a primary condition, the tubes are usually also involved, (salpingo-oöphoritis or tubo-ovarian abscess).

Requires distinction from:	Ovarian tumour Endometriosis Intestinal and urinary tract disorder.

AIDS/HIV

Definition
AIDS = Acquired Immune Deficiency Syndrome. It is characterised by the occurrence of unusual infections or tumours/cancers in individuals who were previously fit and well, i.e.:

- Kaposi's sarcoma
- Primary lymphoma of brain
- *Pneumocystis carinii* pneumonia
- Toxoplasmosis — lungs or CNS
- Cryptosporidiosis — gut — diarrhoea
- Strongyloidosis — gut, CNS or disseminated
- Aspergillosis — CNS or disseminated

- Candidiasis — oesophagus
- Cryptococcosis — CNS, lung or disseminated
- Atypical mycobacteriosis — disseminated
- Cytomegalovirus — lung, CNS, GI tract
- Herpes simplex virus — lung, GIT, disseminated, or chronic mucocutaneous ulcers
- Progressive multifocal leuko-encephalopathy. (Disseminated infection means that lungs and lymph nodes are involved, or other internal organs.)

AIDS is caused by HIV (human immunodeficiency virus).

AIDS is now epidemic in many sub-Saharan countries.

HIV:

Retrovirus (RNA virus + lipid-containing membrane surrounding the capsid + reverse transcriptase [virus can make a DNA copy of its RNA genetic material, facilitating integration into genetic material of host cell, thereby directing host cell to make more RNA viruses])

Has an affinity for T-helper cells

Activated T-helper cells increase viral replication

Viruses liberated by 'budding out' from host cells

Depletion of helper cells — inefficient B lymphocytes, + cytotoxic T cell activity and lymphokine-producing T cell activity are reduced — decreased ability of the immune system to destroy neoplastic and virus-infected cells

Infects glial cells.

Expression of disease may depend on co-factors:

- Genetic predisposition
- Other latent viral infections:
    — CMV
    — EBB
    — HSV
    — Varicella-zoster virus
- Anal intercourse (absorption of semen from rectal mucosa—immunosuppression.)

Origin:	? Species jump from green monkey to human as a result of bite or eating monkey flesh/brains.
Features:	Long incubation period Initial acute febrile illness (sometimes) Many patients complain of: lymphadenopathy sore throat

anorexia
nausea/vomiting
headache
photophobia
diarrhoea
rash (roseola-like)
Acute illness may precede or follow
seroconversion
Antibodies to HIV generally produced 3–6
months (IgG)
Some infected patients fail to form
antibodies
Patients can transmit infection between
infection and seroconversion
Fall in antibody levels seen in advanced
clinical AIDS
AIDS can occur up to 5 years or more
after seroconversion.

AIDS related complex (ARC)

Definition: All the variations in ill-health seen between
asymptomatic seropositive status and
full-blown AIDS sufferers.

ARC = lymphadenopathy—axilla/cervical
fever
night sweats
weight loss
fatigue
+ / – splenomegaly
leukopenia
decrease in T4:T8 cell ratio
thrombocytopenia
oral candidiasis
hairy leukoplakia.

Women at risk of HIV infection
Intravenous drug user
Prostitute
Recent immigrant from high-risk area
Previous transfusion in high-risk area
Partner of i.v. drug user
Partner of bisexual man
Partner from high-risk area
Partner of male with known HIV.

In pregnancy:	No routine screening policy (cf. syphilis screen)
	Offer screening to those at risk (see listing above)
	Pregnancy unlikely to have any long-term adverse effects in asymptomatic women
	Health may deteriorate in immunocompromised woman
	HIV may result in slight reduction in birth weight
	HIV has no significant effect on pregnancy outcome
	In Africa may increase:
	spontaneous abortion
	pre-term labour
	stillbirth
	No increase in congenital abnormalities.

PHLS unlinked anonymous prevalence study (n = 80 000) carried out mainly in antenatal clinics showed prevalence to be <1% amongst non-high-risk women.

Risk of transmission:	Mother to infant <20%
Mode of transmission:	Transplacental
	Genital tract secretions (therefore no scalp electrodes or sampling)
	Breast milk.

Remember transmission to doctors and midwives; the RCOG (1990) advises using barriers:

- gowns
- aprons
- gloves
- masks
- eye protection.

ENDOMETRIOSIS

This is a condition in which the endometrium is found outside the uterine cavity. It is commonly found in the ovaries, pouch of Douglas, vagina or umbilicus, and in scars after gynaecological operations. Bizarre presentations (e.g. cyclical haemoptysis) have been known to occur. Endometrial tissue within the myometrium is called adenomyosis. Adenomyosis is not necessarily associated with endometriosis. Adenomyosis may be produced by the modern technique of endometrial resection.

Aetiology:	? Retrograde menstruation leading to implantation ? Implantation of fragments at operation ? Changes in peritoneal mesothelial cells to endometrial cells.
Features:	Common in Europe and USA Rare in Negroes Common in nulliparous women Pelvic pain Dysmenorrhoea Menorrhagia Frequent periods Dyspareunia Infertility Pelvic pressure symptoms Uterine retroversion Thickening of the utero-sacral ligaments Nodules in the pouch of Douglas Ovarian enlargement and tenderness (Chocolate cysts) Painful defaecation.
Diagnosis:	History Examination Laparoscopy ⎫ with confirmatory Laporotomy ⎭ histopathology, although appearance characteristic.
Treatment: Medical:	Continuous progestogen (e.g. norethisterone) Continuous danazol (an anti-gonadotrophic agent) GnRH analogues, e.g. buserelin.
Surgical:	Diathermy of endometriomata (can be done down a laparoscope) Excision of endometriomata TAH + BSO.

Neoplasia and related disorders

Neoplasia may be:

- congenital or acquired
- benign or malignant
- solid or cystic.

CONGENITAL

Vulva:

Teratoma
Haemangioma.

Vagina:

'Adenosis' (mothers given oestrogens during pregnancy)
Cysts of Gartner's duct.

Cervix:

Mesonephric cysts
Sarcoma botryoides.

Uterus

Nil.

Fallopian tubes:

Fimbrial cysts.

Ovaries:

Parovarian cysts
Hydatid of Morgagni
Wolffian remnants.

ACQUIRED (BENIGN OR MALIGNANT)

Vulva

The following list covers 'tumours' in the widest possible sense, including lesions which cause enlargement of the vulva.

Benign:

Oedema
Haematoma
Bartholin's cyst/abscess

Sebaceous cyst
Lipoma
Granuloma
Haemangioma (senile; cf. congenital)
Lymphangioma
Fibroma
Neurofibroma
Seborrhoeic keratosis.

Management: Excision if necessary.

Malignant (carcinoma of the vulva):
                               A rare condition — 4% of all primary
                                   genital cancers
                               85–90% are squamous carcinomas
                               Others are undifferentiated
                               Occurs in postmenopausal women
                               Long history of pruritus and bloodstained
                                   discharge
                               Association with vulvar dystrophies
                               Early lesions resemble
                                   infection/inflammation
                               Late lesions ulcerated or polypoid
                               Commonly on anterior part of labia
                                   majora
                               Biopsy essential.

Unusual cancers: Tumours of Bartholin's gland
                               Malignant melanoma
                               Rodent ulcer
                               Carcinoma of urethra

Management: Biopsy
                               Result benign — continued observation
                               Result dysplastic — may be observed
                                   with repeat biopsy, or
                                   simply vulvectomy
                               Result malignant — radical vulvectomy ±
                                   radiotherapy to remaining groin and
                                   pelvic nodes.

VULVAR DYSTROPHIES

The term vulvar dystrophy includes atrophic and hypertrophic
lesions, which produce circumscribed or widespread white skin. In

atrophic conditions the skin is white because there are few blood vessels, in hypertrophy the whiteness occurs because the thickened epidermis blocks the normal pink colour. An inflammatory infiltrate is present. Dysplasia and cancer can develop in both types of lesion. Suspicious areas must be biopsied. Evaluate lesions colposcopically if possible.

Treatment: Atrophic lesions: topical testosterone
                            ointment
                          Hypertrophic lesions: topical steroids
                          Topical oestrogens most useful for
                            pre-menarchal patient. Both lesions
                            symptomatically improved with
                            vaseline.
                          Steroids aggravate atrophic lesions, but
                            may give good symptomatic relief.
                          Simple vulvectomy occasionally required
                            for chronic pruritus.
                          Regular review necessary.
                          (May be stress related in younger women).

CARCINOMA OF THE VAGINA

Very rare, 1–2% of genital tract cancers.

Presents with: Painless bleeding
                          Pain
                          Swelling
                          An ulcerated or polypoid tumour
                          Cachexia (late).

Types (primary):   Squamous (the majority)
                          Adenocarcinoma (clear cell)
                          Melanoma ⎤
                          Sarcoma   ⎦ rare

Secondaries from: Uterus
                          Cervix
                          Ovary
                          Bladder
                          Urethra
                          Rectum
                          Bowel
                          Vulva
                          Choriocarinoma.

Treatment:
This is difficult due to the proximity of the rectum and bladder.
Mainstay is radiotheraphy.

Surgery: Vaginectomy
                             Pelvic exenteration.

NB Vaginal cancers spreading to other genital structures are
    considered to be tumours of that structure.
    To diagnose vaginal cancer the lesion must be clearly confined to
    the vagina.

CERVICAL NEOPLASIA

Benign 'tumours' of   Nabothian cysts (blocked mucous glands)
the cervix: Mesonephric cysts (Wolffian duct
                                 remnants)
                             Polyps (cause abnormal bleeding; remove)
                             Papillomas (95% benign; excise or
                                 cauterise)
                             Fibroids (uncommon)
                             Endometrioma (unusual; rarely large; excise
                                 or cauterise).

Carcinoma-in-situ
Cervical intra-epithelial neoplasia are graded 1, 2, and 3:

- CIN 1 = mild dysplasia/abnormality
- CIN 2 = moderate dysplasia
- CIN 3 = severe dysplasia + CIS (carcinoma-in-situ).

Cervical dysplasia is considered to be a pre-malignant condition. It is
often asymptomatic, but may present 'classically' with post-coital
bleeding, and also inter-menstrual bleeding and discharge. Detected
by cervical cytology, BUT note 11–15% false negative rate!

Treatment
This is by local   Cone biopsy
ablation: Radical cautery
                              Cryocautery
                              Laser
                              Hysterectomy (abdominal or vaginal).

Guidelines on repeat smears are laid out in Figure 16.

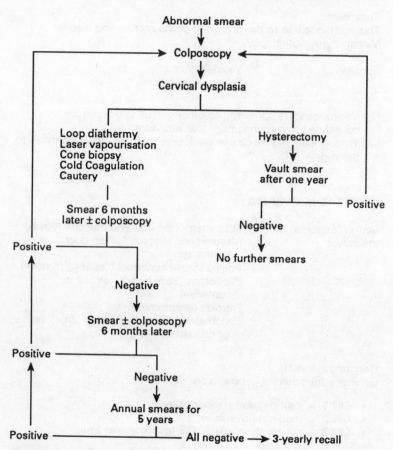

Fig. 16 Guidelines on repeat smears

Carcinoma of the cervix

This condition is associated with intercourse, human papillomavirus infection, early age of first intercourse, multiparity, promiscuity, non-barrier methods of contraception, smoking and low socio-economic groups. It causes 2000–2500 deaths per annum in England and Wales.

The previously held theory of a low incidence of this condition in the partners of circumcised males is no longer valid.

Associations with the pill may reflect usage by young women starting intercourse as teenagers, with multiple partners, in social classes 4 and 5.

| Cell types: | Squamous carcinoma | 95% |
| | Adenocarcinoma | 5% |

Features:
Early lesions (micro-invasive and occult) may be asymptomatic, detected by smear, colposcopy or biopsy.
  Biopsy is essential. A micro-invasive or invasive cancer may lie below epithelium with CIN3/CIS.

Symptoms:	Post-coital bleeding
	Inter-menstrual bleeding
	Postmenopasual bleeding
	Offensive bloodstained vaginal discharge
	Pelvic discomfort and pain
	Cachexia.

Symptoms due to involvement of adjacent organs:	Tenesmus and diarrhoea
	Fistula
	Haematuria
	Renal failure (ureters)
	Abdominal distension and vomiting (small bowel)
	Referred nerve pain.

Management:	History
	Examination
	Examination under anaesthesia with wedge or cone biopsy
	CXR IVU lymphangiogram after confirmation of diagnosis
	MSU
	FBC + ESR
	U + E creatinine clearance
	LFTs
	Pelvic ultrasound scan
	Bone scan in poorly differentiated lesions in young women
	CAT scans and MRI scans may be useful

Staging
The purpose of the above investigations is to stage the tumour, i.e. to assess how advanced it is and to detect metastases.
  Treatment varies according to the stage.
  The aim should be to give the maximum appropriate treatment with the minimum of side-effects/complications.

FIGO staging

Stage 0:	Carcinoma-in-situ/CIN 3.
Stage 1:	Confined to the cervix; Ia microinvasive; 1b others.
Stage 2:	Beyond cervix but not reaching pelvic side walls Involving upper 2/3rds vagina.
Stage 3:	Cancer extends to pelvic side wall or to lower 1/3rd vagina or there is hydronephrosis or a non-functioning kidney.
Stage 4:	Cancer extends beyond pelvis Involves bladder or rectal mucosa Distant metastases.

Surgery and radiotherapy: both have complications, and combined treatment produces greater morbidity/mortality.

Hence the need to stage accurately this disease in order to administer the single most appropriate therapy.

Treatment:

Stage 1:	1a Microinvasive lesions 5mm or less may be treated by cone biopsy or simple hysterectomy 1b Wertheim's hysterectomy or radiotherapy; surgery better for young women; results the same.
Stage 2:	Radiotherapy + or – chemotherapy.
Stage 3:	Radiotherapy + or – chemotherapy.
Stage 4:	Radiotherapy + chemotherapy Symptomatic and palliative treatment.

Chemotherapy: useful in poorly differentiated tumours. The survival analysis of patients treated for squamous cells carcinoma of the cervix is illustrated in Figure 17.

Regular follow-up is mandatory, ideally in a joint gynaecology/radiotherapy clinic.

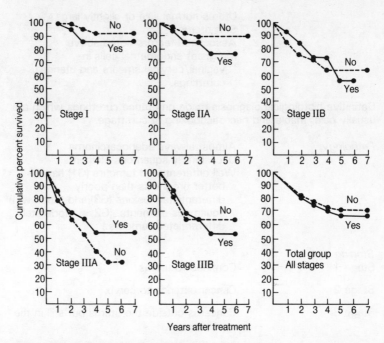

Years after treatment

Fig. 17 Survival curves of patients treated for squamous cell carcinoma of the cervix. Curves for Stages I, IIA, IIB, IIIA and IIIB and all stages combined are shown. Patients who had lymphadenectomy added to their treatment are represented by solid curves. The broken curves are for patients who had radiation treatment only. (Reproduced with permission from Ratledge)

CARCINOMA OF THE ENDOMETRIUM

Used to be much less common than cervical cancer, but now more common. Approximately 3% of women will develop the disease if they live beyond 50 years. Mean age 60–70 years. Aetiology unknown.

Associated factors:	Obesity
	Diabetes mellitus
	Hypertension
	Low parity/nulliparity
	Unopposed continuous oestrogen therapy.
Features:	Postmenopausal bleeding
	Abnormal peri-menopausal bleeding
	Vaginal discharge

Uterus normal size or slightly large
Soft uterus
Associated factors noted above
Malignant endometrial cells in
vaginal/cervical smears and uterine
curettings.

Definitive histological diagnosis made on uterine curettings which are usually pale, friable and necrotic looking at curettage.

Pathology   Almost always adenocarcinoma
Occasionally squamous elements
Well differentiated tumours (G1) have a
better prognosis than poorly
differentiated lesions (G3) and those with
squamous elements. (G2 = moderately
differentiated tumours.)

Staging
Stage 1:   Confined to uterus.

Stage 2:   Cancer extends to cervix

Stage 3:   Cancer is outside the uterus but still in the
pelvis.

Stage 4:   Spread into bladder or rectum or distant
metastases.

Management
Surgery: Total abdominal hysterectomy + bilateral
salpingo-oöphorectomy + cuff of vagina
(traditional).

Radiotherapy to vault by means of ovoids: External radiotherapy depends on site of lesion and degree of penetration of myometrium. (Fundal lesions may spread to the nodes draining the ovaries.)

Progestogen therapy: not of proven benefit.
NB Endometrial (cystic glandular) hyperplasia and adenomatous (microglandular) hyperplasia may both become malignant.

FIBROIDS

Leiomyoma (smooth muscle tumours) contain fibrous tissue as well and have a psuedo-capsule. They are very common and influenced by oestrogen. Caucasian women often present over the age of 30 years. Large fibroids can occur at a much younger age in negroes.

Pathology:	Multiple Capsule of compressed myometrium Subserous + / − pedicle Intramural Submucous + / − pedicle Cervical Produce irregular uterine enlargement Degenerate.
Types of degeneration *(favourite examiners* *question):*	Atrophy (postmenopausal) Hyaline (most large fibroids) Cystic (in hyaline areas) Calcification (postmenopausal large fibroids) Red (infarction, especially in pregnancy) Fatty Sarcomatous (malignant change; rare).

Pedunculated fibroids can undergo torsion.

Symptoms:	Often none
	Heavy periods
	Painful periods
	Frequent periods
	Lower abdominal swelling
	Pelvic pain/discomfort
	May be associated with infertility
	Pressure symptoms:
	    stress incontinence
	    urge incontinence
	    frequency
	    rectal pressure
	Varicose veins ⎫
	Piles ⎬ Symptoms of
	Ankle oedema ⎭ venous obstruction.

Fibroids can impact in the pelvis causing acute retention of urine.

Signs:	Enlarged irregular uterus Smooth swellings Generally non-tender.
Diagnostic aids:	EUA + D&C Ultrasound scan X-ray shows calcified fibroids.
Treatment:	Nil (if asymptomatic) Hysterectomy Myomectomy if women wishes to conserve fertility.

Fibroids in pregnancy: May cause:
pain (red degeneration)
abnormal lie
malpresentation
obstruct labour
uterine inertia
postpartum haemorrhage. — *due to inefficient uterine contraction*

Never remove fibroids in pregnancy or at caesarean section. There may be fatal haemorrhage.

TROPHOBLASTIC DISEASE

This condition is 10 times more common in the Far East than in Europe. Remember that normal trophoblast is invasive. There are benign and malignant forms of the disease.

Hydatidiform mole (benign end of the spectrum)

Diagnostic features: Rapid uterine enlargement
Large for dates uterus
Excessive nausea and vomiting
Early onset of PET
Absent fetal heart
Snowstorm appearance on ultrasound
scan
Uterine discomfort due to stretching
Grape-like vesicles passed
High urine HCG titres
Bilateral ovarian cysts (theca lutein) in half
the cases.

Distinguish from: Multiple pregnancy
Hydraminos
Fibroids.

Pathology/Aetiology
Cystic degeneration of chorionic villi
Occurs during first 18 weeks of pregnancy
Cause unknown; chromosomes XX — both from sperm.
May cause: Haemorrhage
Infection
Uterine rupture.

Up to 20% of cases become malignant, i.e. develop into choriocarcinoma.

Treatment

Empty uterus by: Suction evacuation
Uterine stimulation (Syntocinon;
    prostaglandins)
Hysterectomy.

Curettage 7–10 days later, probably of little benefit.
Careful follow-up.
Patient avoids pregnancy (pill after HCG levels become normal).

Regular: CXR
Urinary HCG levels
β sub-unit HCG levels (serum).

Residual/persistent disease is treated with chemotherapy.

Choriocarcinoma (malignant end of the spectrum)

Curable
Early identification and treatment essential
Chemotherapy = methotrexate (folic acid antagonist)
Metastasises to:

- lungs
- liver
- brain
- vagina
- kidney

Best treated at specialist referral centre. Metastases may be
removed.

OVARIAN TUMOURS

Ovarian tumours may be benign or malignant, primary or secondary,
solid or cystic; most benign tumours have cystic elements.
Remember the congenital cysts at the start of the chapter.

Benign

Cysts are usually   Graafian follicle
physiological   Corpus luteum

or retention cysts   Follicular cyst (from atretic follicles).

Endometriosis causes   Chocolate cysts.

Other benign tumours: Mucinous cystadenoma
                         (can be massive)
                         Serous cystadenoma
                         Dermoid cyst
                         Fibroma (can cause hydrothorax —
                         Meig's syndrome).

Symptoms: May be none
               Pain with tortion, rupture or bleeding
               (may mimic ectopic pregnancy)
               Swelling
               Pressure effects
               Urinary retention
               Acute abdomen (through rupture).

Signs: Pelvic swelling
            Smooth
            Often mobile
            Dull to percussion
            Cystic on ultrasound.

Treatment: Generally any cyst >5 cm diameter should
                be removed if it does not go
                spontaneously. Smaller cyst should be kept
                under review.
                   In pregnancy ovarian cysts are best
                removed at about 16 weeks' gestation.
                   Interest is being shown in the
                development of ultrasound screening of the
                ovaries for the early detection of ovarian
                cancer, using colour Doppler to detect
                abnormal vasculature.

OVARIAN CARCINOMA

Ovarian carcinoma kills >3000 women in England and Wales per
year, and about 2% of women in their 50s and 60s will die of the
disease. Late presentation is common, many patients presenting with
advanced Stage 3 disease. Ovarian cancer is primary or secondary,
solid or cystic.

Aetiology: Unknown
                Malignant change in a benign lesion.
                Possibly more common in single women.

Primary tumour types:	Mucinous cystadenocarcinoma ⎫ most common — epithelial tumours
	Serous Cystadenocarcinoma ⎬
	Endometrioid
	Granulosa cell
	Dysgerminoma.

Secondary tumours from: Breast
Stomach
Colon (by direct and lymphatic spread).

Krukenberg tumours are secondary gastrointestinal tumours.

FIGO staging

Stage 1: Confined to ovaries:
1a one ovary, no ascites
1b two ovaries, no ascites
1c one or two ovaries with ascites or tumour on ovarian capsule.

Stage 2: One or two ovaries with extension to the pelvis.

Stage 3: Widespread intra-peritoneal metastases (omentum commonly involved) or positive retroperitoneal nodes.

Stage 4: Distant metastases.

Features: Late onset of symptoms
Adnexal swelling
Abdominal swelling/distension (tumour + / − ascites)
Pressure symptoms (see Fibroids)
Pain
Cachexia
Bowel symptoms (very important: any woman over 40 years of age with GI symptoms — think ovarian cancer)
May be associated with a second primary (often bowel)
Often referred from physicians or general surgeons, having presented with non-gynaecological symptoms.

Investigations:	FBC
	U + E
	LFTs
	CA 125
	Creatinine
	MSU
	CXR
	IVU (optional)
	Barium enema (optional)
	Scans are unhelpful as they have no effect on the ultimate management.
Treatment:	Surgical 'debulking' for all stages if possible
	'Debulk' = total abdominal hysterectomy + bilateral salpingo-oöphorectomy + omentectomy + any other tumour greater than 2 cm diameter
	Adjuvant therapy — chemotherapy for lesions that have spread beyond one ovary with no malignant cells in peritoneal fluid, i.e. 1ai; CA 125 levels used to assess response
	Regular follow-up is essential
	Second-look surgery does not improve survival (CAN monitor) with CA 125 levels).

BASIC MANAGEMENT OF TERMINAL GYNAECOLOGICAL CANCER

Terminal care for the gynaecological cancer patient is the same as that for any cancer patient, but cancer of the female genital tract is often complicated by fistula, whether due to the disease process or as a complication of radiotherapy.

Terminal care may/should include the following:

- terminal admissions average 2 weeks (teaching hospitals admit 2% of UK deaths)
- pain relief without sedation
- avoid constipation
- control vomiting and nausea
- companionship
- occupy the mind
- psychological support

- good all-round communication
- stop chemotherapy?
- arrange residential care as required
- symptomatic relief — drain ascites — tap pleural effusion
- steroids to improve sense of well-being and help bone pain
- nerve/epidural blocks.

Retroversion, genital prolapse and gynaecological urology

RETROVERSION OF THE UTERUS

Uterine retroversion is not invariably pathological. It is a variant of the normal uterine position, and it is often asymptomatic.

Retroversion: The axis of the body of the uterus is directed to the hollow of the sacrum. The cervix points anteriorly.

Retroflexion: The axis of the body of the uterus is directed to the hollow of the sacrum BUT the axis of the cervix remains in the normal axis.

Causes
Congenital:
Acquired:

Adhesions ——— Pelvic infection ⎫ Fixed

Endometriosis ⎬ Retroversion

Fibroids
Occurs *during* uterine prolapse.

Features: May be none
Dyspareunia
?Subfertility
Incarceration of gravid uterus with acute
    urinary retention
Incarceration of gravid uterus with abortion
    (rare) (historical)

Management: Treat cause
Correct position with a Hodge pessary
    (unusual in modern practice)
Ventrosuspension/shortening of the round
    ligaments (becoming an unusual
    procedure).

Caution: Any pelvic surgery can cause adhesions
                         and tubal damage with subsequent
                         infertility.

Incarceration of the gravid uterus requires catheterisation of the
patient, and may require anteversion of the uterus under general
anaesthesia.

GENITAL PROLAPSE

The walls of the vagina, vaginal fornices and uterus can prolapse. A
protrusion such as an enterocoele can be considered as a true hernia.

Types: Cystocoele
                         Urethrocoele
                         Rectocoele
                         Enterocoele
                         Uterine prolapse (cervical/vault descent)

Definitions

Cystocoele: Prolapse of the posterior bladder wall and
                         trigone and anterior vaginal wall. Usually
                         occurs with an urethrocoele.

Urethrocoele: Prolapse of the urethra, usually with the
                         bladder neck.

Rectocoele: Prolapse of the anterior rectal wall with the
                         posterior vaginal wall. A recto-vaginal
                         'hernia'.

Enterocoele: Hernia of the pouch of Douglas through the
                         posterior vaginal fornix, containing small
                         bowel.

Uterine prolapse: An abnormal descent of the uterus through
                         the vagina.

Aetiology

All prolapse share a common aetiology: weakness of structures
supporting the pelvic organs.

Supporting structures: Pelvic floor (levator ani + perineal body)
                         Ligaments + connective tissue of pelvic
                              fascia
                         Cardinal ligaments
                         Uterosacral ligaments
                         Pubo-cervical fascia.

Weakening factors:	Childbirth (? episiotomy protects)
	Postmenopausal atrophy
	Raised intra-abdominal pressure:
	obesity
	chronic cough
	chronic constipation.

Features

Cystocoele and urethrocoele:	Vaginal fullness
	'Something falling out' or 'a lump down below'
	Incomplete bladder emptying
	Stress incontinence
	Need to push lump up to pass urine
	Soft reducible mass in introitus
	Increased bulge with straining, reduces on lying.

Rectocoele:	Difficult defaecation
	Vaginal fullness
	'Something falling out' — reduces on lying
	Soft reducible mass posterior vaginal wall
	Thin perineum — skin, no muscle.

Enterocoele:	Vaginal discomfort
	'Something falling down'
	Bulging mass posterior fornix
	Associated with uterine prolapse/post TAH and post colposuspension
	Post menopausal women
	Simultaneous rectal and vaginal examination distinguishes from rectocoele.

Uterine prolapse:	Firm mass lower vagina
	Cervix through introitus
	Inside-out vagina
	Vaginal fullness
	'Something coming down'
	Sacral back-ache
	Ulceration causing post menopausal bleeding.

Degrees:	1°: descent in vagina ⎤ spontaneous 2°: descent in introitus ⎦ reduction on on lying down
	3°: descent outside vagina; no spontaneous reduction.

Remember: Genital prolapse is best examined with Sim's speculum, in the left lateral position.

Management:	History
	General examination
	Gynaecological examination and cervical
	smear.

Treatment
Conservative or surgical.

Conservative:	None if asymptomatic
	Vaginal pessary (permanent or temporary):
	ring or shelf
	Pelvic floor exercises.

Surgery:	Anterior repair
	Posterior repair
	Vaginal hysterectomy
	Manchester repair.

Pregnancy not contraindicated after a repair.
Vaginal delivery probably unwise after a successful repair for stress
incontinence. Therefore delay surgery until family completed.

GYNAECOLOGICAL UROLOGY

Urinary incontinence
This is the involuntary loss of urine; intermittent or continuous.

Types:	Enuresis
	True incontinence
	Stress incontinence
	Urgency incontinence
	Overflow incontinence.

Enuresis

Definition:	Uncontrolled emptying of bladder at night
	Normal up to 3 years of age
	Investigate after 6 years for physiological,
	anatomical or psychological abnormality.

True incontinence

| *Congenital:* | Ectopic ureter |
| | Ectopia vesicae. |

Acquired:	Trauma to urethra/bladder neck
	Senile dementia
	Disseminated sclerosis

Paraplegia
Fistula:
  uretero-vaginal (iatrogenic or due to
    malignant disease)
  vesico-vaginal (iatrogenic, obstructed
    labour, malignant disease, DXT).

Stress incontinence

Definition: The involuntary loss of urine with a sudden
  rise in intra-abdominal pressure,
  Common; about 50% of all women
  >45 years
  Parous.

Aetiology: Loss of support at urethro-vesical junction;
  bladder base descent, resulting in a
  shorter, wider urethra; less resistance to
  flow.

Causes: All causes of genital prolapse above.

Urgency incontinence

Definition: Urgent desire to void urine followed by the
  involuntary loss of urine
  Due to detrusor instability
  Can occur with stress incontinence.

Causes: Infection
  Atrophic/menopausal changes
  Irradiation
  Calculi
  Diverticula
  DS
  Urethritis
  Neurogenic bladder.

Overflow incontinence

Definitions: Overdistension of the bladder resulting in a
  dribbling incontinence.

Aetiology: Urethral stenosis
  After vaginal surgery
  Postpartum
  Loss of bladder sensation due to age or
    neurological disorder
  Incarcerated pelvic mass.

Diagnosis of incontinence (see the flow-chart; Fig. 18)

The history is the most important factor in making the correct diagnosis.

Examination

Special investigations.

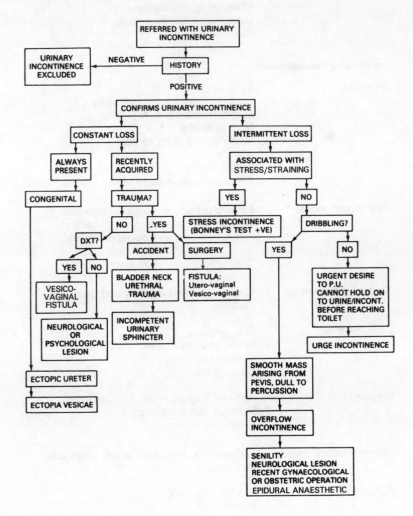

Fig. 18 Diagnosis of incontinence

Examination:	With a full bladder Sim's speculum Bonney's test.
Special tests:	Pyridium instilled into bladder for fistula Methylene blue i.v. for ureteric fistula MSU IVU Micturating cystogram Cystometry/urodynamics Cystoscopy.

Treatment/management

Enuresis:	Exclude UTI Exclude renal tract abnormality Empty bladder before retiring No late drinks Wake during night to void Alarms Imipramine Support + encouragement.
True incontinence:	Ectopic ureter — surgical correction Ectopia vesicae — surgical correction Fistula — closure or urinary diversion Senility — catheter.
Stress incontinence:	Exclude UTI and urgency and pelvic masses.
Conservative:	Ring pessary Pelvic floor exercises Weight reduction Oestrogens.
Surgical:	Anterior vaginal repair (colporrhaphy) Remove pelvic tumours Colposuspension.
Urgency incontinence:	Exclude UTI, neurological and urological abnormality.
Surgery:	NEVER indicated Bladder drill Anti-cholinergic drugs *may* help.

Overflow incontinence: Catheterise
Rest bladder
Correction of stenosis
Permanent catheter for neurological deficit.

Cystitis
Inflammation of the bladder (acute or chronic). Much more common in females than males.

Common causative   Esch. coli
organisms: Enterobacter
Klebsiella
Strep. faecalis
Proteus
Pseudomonas
Don't forget TB.

Symptoms: Dysuria (burning/painful micturition)
Urgency
Frequency
Pain — supra-pubic and low back
Haematuria — occasionally gross
Fever.

Aetiology: Bacterial infection: poor hygiene sexual
intercourse
instrumentation
Radiation
Fistula — colo-vesical.

Investigation: MSU — microscopy, culture and sensitivity
Positive = >5 WBC/HPF or >10^5
organisms/HPF
Recurrent cystitis requires:
IVU ± renal ultrasound scan
cystoscopy

IVU and cystoscopy are mandatory when there has been haematuria. Urine cytology is useful.

Treatment   Correct aetiological factor if possible
Education
Antibiotics
High fluid intake
Mist. pot. cit. or pyridium for dysuria
Post-coital antibiotic prophylaxis
Long-term antibiotic prophylaxis.

Urethritis
Inflammation of the urethra, acute or chronic.

Common causative organism — Gonococcus
Non-gonococcal   *Chlamydia trachomatis*
(non-specific) urethritis: T-strain mycoplasma
                        Corynebacterium.

Symptoms: Dysuria
                        Frequency
                        (Abscess may occasionally form).

Aetiology: Sexual intercourse
                        Instrumentation.

Investigation: Swabs — urethral + cervical
                        (Special swabs and transport medium for
                            chlamydia)
                        Serological tests for syphilis
                        MSU.

Treatment:
VD suspected: Refer to special clinic
                        Rapid identification of organism
                        Contact tracing.

Gonorrhoea: A penicillin + probenecid 1–2 g orally to
                            block renal excretion of penicillin
                        Tetracycline for resistant strains.

NSU: Tetracycline/oxytetracycline/ofloxacin
                        Avoid alcohol for 2 weeks

Haematuria
Blood in the urine. Colours urine red or brown depending on the
amount of blood and the urine pH. Slight haematuria may produce no
colour change, being detected by microscopy.

Painless: Renal
                        Vesical
                        Casts = glomerulonephritis
                        No casts, think of renal or bladder
                            tumour
                        Stones
                        Polycystic kidney.

Painful: Stone (renal colic)
                                        Infection — cystitis
                                                    pyelonephritis.

Remember schistosomiasis in immigrant patients.

Urethral stricture
Congenital or acquired
Acquired: Trauma — obstetric   } peri-urethral
                                                  coital   } fibrosis.

Symptoms: Dysuria
                                        Slow stream
                                        Infection.

Special tests: Urethroscopy
                                        Cysto-urethrography.

Treatment: Urethral dilatation.

Urethral caruncle
Small, red, fleshy, sensitive 'growth' at *posterior* margin of the
external urinary meatus
Single
Comprises vascular granulation tissue + thin stratified transitional or
squamous epithelium
May be infected; probably caused by infection.

Symptoms: Bleeding: PMB or haematuria
                                        Dysuria
                                        Frequency
                                        Pain
                                        Urgency
                                        Dyspareunia
                                        Malignant change (very rare).

Treatment: Excision
                                        Cautery
                                        Oestrogen cream.

Urethral mucosal prolapse
May be confused with caruncle. May be distinguished from caruncle
because it surrounds the external urethral meatus. It may be present
in children.

Treatment: Excision.

Urethral diverticulum

Usually found in the mid-portion of the urethra, and the patient is usually over middle-age. They lie in the mid-line.

Cause:	Rupture of para-urethral (Wolffian) remnant Injury.
Symptoms:	Para-urethral swelling Dysuria Purulent urethral discharge Dyspareunia.

Distinguish between:	Urethrocoele — a mid-line, reducible
	    swelling
	Abscess of Skene's gland — opens at
	    urethral margin
	Cyst of Gartner's duct — no urethral
	    connection.

Urethral carcinoma

Rare
Squamous or transitional cell; occasionally adenocarcinoma.

Symptoms:	Haematuria Local mass.
Lymphatic drainage:	Lower urethra — inguinal glands Upper urethra — obturator glands and internal iliac glands.
Treatment:	Radiotherapy Surgery.

The prognosis is poor.

Pyelonephritis

A diffuse, often bilateral, pyogenic infection of the kidney. Clinically, infection of the renal pelvis cannot be distinguished from infection of the renal parenchyma. Extremely serious for the pregnant patient. Associated with pre-term labour and fetal mortality.

Aetiology:	Urinary stasis Bacterial invasion Infection *Esch. coli* in 85% of infections Catheterisation Haematogenous spread (most common with staphylococcal bacteraemia).

Symptoms:	Fever Rigor Pain/tenderness in renal angle Dysuria Haematuria Frequency Urgency Nausea + vomiting (± Uterine contractions).
Investigations:	MSU = pyuria organisms > 100 000/ml on culture FBC + ESR ⎫ IVU ⎬ if haematuria. Cystoscopy ⎭
Treatment	Fluids — oral/i.v. Antibiotics (after MSU) MSU at regular intervals In pregnancy — long-term antibiotics/antiseptics.

NB Recurrent infection is either a relapse (the same organism), or a re-infection (different organism).

Relapsing infections:	Renal source May require parenteral antibiotic.
Re-infection:	Bladder infections usually.

Endocrine and related disorders

AMENORRHOEA

Definition: Absence of menstruation for 6 months or more.

The distinction between primary and secondary amenorrhoea is of little use clinically as the causes overlap (but note that secondary amenorrhoea implies that there has been an intact functioning genital tract). The term 'post-pill amenorrhoea' should also be avoided since not only is it uncertain whether the condition exists as a discrete entity, but also its use as a 'diagnosis' may divert attention from more serious causes.

Oligomenorrhoea is defined as menstruation occurring at intervals of greater than 6 weeks, up to 6 months. In practice it is not usefully considered as a separate entity, since the causes of oligomenorrhoea are in effect those of amenorrhoea.

Incidence: The incidence of amenorrhoea in women or reproductive years is approximately 1–2%.

Causes

Physiological: Pre-menarche and post menopausally Pregnancy and often during lactation.

Pathological:
i.e. occurring in the absence of pregnancy in a woman of child-bearing age (16 years the upper limit of normal for the menarche, to 40 years the lower limit for the menopause).

Anatomical (1% of all cases):
                           Congenital, e.g. vaginal atresia
                           Acquired, e.g. endometrial fibrosis
                           (Asherman's syndrome).

Endocrine (99% of all cases):

Primary endocrine organ failure (12%):
primary hypothalamic failure
primary pituitary failure
primary ovarian failure
Hyperprolactinaemia (20%):
pituitary tumours
drug induced hyperprolactinaemia, e.g.
phenothiazines
hypothyroidism (causes raised TSH).
Polycystic ovarian syndrome
Miscellaneous (rare — ? 2% in all):
thyroid disease
diabetes mellitus
Hypothalamic disorders (60%):
feed-back disorders (often with marked
psychological element, e.g. anorexia
nervosa)
cycle initiation defect.

Investigations

History and clinical examination:
Especially for:

Weight loss — psychiatric disorders
Symptoms/signs suggestive of thyroid
disease
Drug history
Hirsutism/virilism
Genital tract abnormality (e.g.
obstruction due to imperforate hymen).
NB Cryptomenorrhoea is concealed
menstruation due to an imperforate
hymen.

Endocrine investigations:

Serum prolactin (if raised, XR (or CT scan)
sella turcica) + visual field assessment
Progesterone challenge test: if no
withdrawal bleed, proceed to combined
oestrogen and progesterone challenge
Serum FSH/LH assay
Thyroid function test
Clomiphene response if infertility an
associated problem.

These investigations, and how they are used to arrive at a diagnosis, are summarised in the flow chart (Fig. 19).

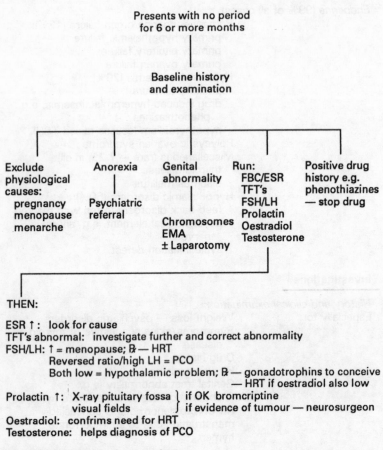

Presents with no period
for 6 or more months

Baseline history
and examination

**Exclude
physiological
causes:**
pregnancy
menopause
menarche

Anorexia

Psychiatric
referral

**Genital
abnormality**

Chromosomes
EMA
± Laparotomy

Run:
FBC/ESR
TFT's
FSH/LH
Prolactin
Oestradiol
Testosterone

**Positive drug
history e.g.
phenothiazines
— stop drug**

THEN:

ESR ↑ : look for cause
TFT's abnormal: investigate further and correct abnormality
FSH/LH: ↑ = menopause; ℞ — HRT
         Reversed ratio/high LH = PCO
         Both low = hypothalamic problem; ℞ — gonadotrophins to conceive
                                              — HRT if oestradiol also low
Prolactin ↑ : X-ray pituitary fossa ⎫ if OK bromcriptine
              visual fields   ⎭ if evidence of tumour — neurosurgeon
Oestradiol: confirms need for HRT
Testosterone: helps diagnosis of PCO

Fig. 19 Investigation of amenorrhoea

Added to these, chromosome studies for the karyotype may be
useful

Management

Depends on: (i) The cause of the amenorrhoea
                       (ii) Whether infertility is an associated
                       problem.

If infertility is not an associated problem, contraception will usually be
required in addition to the treatment outlined below in the table.

Table 4. Treatment of amenorrhoea

Diagnosis	Treatment	
	Infertility is a problem	Infertility not a problem
Primary hypothalamic/pituitary failure	Gonadotrophins (beware over-stimulation)	Oestrogen replacement therapy
Primary ovarian failure	Pregnancy only possible with ovum or embryo donation at an IVF unit	Oestrogen replacement

Hyperprolactinaemia	No difference in treatment:
	  Drug induced — stop drug
	  Tumours — small — bromocriptine
	            — large — (especially if pregnant) pituitary ablation as tumour may grow rapidly. Visual fields must be checked regularly	

Primary hypothyroidism	Thyroxine	
Polycystic ovarian syndrome	Clomiphene (Wedge resection of ovary)	Virilising tumour — excision Hirsutism — OCP ($\uparrow$ SHBG) or cyproterone acetate and oestrogen
'Hypothalamic disorders'	Clomiphene Gonadotrophins Psychiatric referral	Anorexia nervosa and related disorders

MENOPAUSE

By definition, the last menstrual period.
   Average in UK — 51 years.
   The climacteric is the time of life around the menopause 'when the vital force begins to decline' (*Oxford English Dictionary*).
   The primary event of the menopause (and climacteric) is ovarian failure resulting in decreased oestrogen production: it is this decrease in oestrogen which results in the physiological and symptomatic effects of the menopause.

Physiological consequences of the menopause:	Amenorrhoea Vulval and vaginal atrophy Thinning of the endometrium Body of the uterus shrinks relative to the cervix Osteoporosis Breast atrophy Urinary tract atrophy.

Symptoms:	Hot flushes
	Atrophic vulvo-vaginitis
	Urinary disturbances
	Psychiatric disturbances
	Increased incidence of ischaemic heart disease
	Increased incidence of fractures.

Clinically useful symptoms suggestive of the climacteric:
Any of the above may indicate the presence of the climacteric, but in particular:

Hot flushes and sweats
Lengthening menstrual cycles
Mood and sleep disturbances.

Post-menopausal hormone pattern:	FSH greatly increased (can be used diagnostically)
	LH moderately raised
	Oestrogen levels fall
	Prolactin levels fall
	Progesterone levels fall.

Possible treatment(s) for menopausal symptoms (treatment is not always indicated):

Oestrogens:	Only hot flushes and vulvo-vaginitis are known to respond
	Osteoporosis may be prevented (but not reversed)
	Oestrogen therapy is not without risk: therapy should be cyclical and be combined with 12 days' progestogen/progesterone to reduce risk of endometrial carcinoma
	Therapy is contraindicated in a few conditions (including oestrogen-dependent tumours and acute liver disease).

Surgery (rare) e.g. dilatation of the lower urethra; excision of urethral caruncle.

Sympathetic and understanding approach, but consider psychiatric referral if FSH/LH not menopausal or symptoms do not respond to HRT.

Premature menopause
Rare
Pathophysiological event is primary ovarian failure occurring before age of 40 years.

Diagnosis:	FSH greatly increased (with moderate LH increase)
	Ovarian biopsy may be performed to exclude 'resistant' ovaries
	Screen for auto-immune disease (increased incidence).

HIRSUTISM

Causes and pathophysiology: see p. 27

Investigation:	Plasma testosterone and SHBG
	Serum FSH/LH assay
	21st day progesterone (to confirm/refute ovulation) if having a cycle
	Other endocrinological investigations as indicated:
	human growth hormone assay
	urinary free cortisol
	plasma cortisol and ACTH
	pituitary fossa XR.
Treatment:	Tumours — excision
	Glucocorticoids for adrenal cortex disturbances
	OCP — causes increased SHBG which mops up testosterone
	Cyproterone acetate — thought to act directly on hair follicles but is teratogenic and must therefore be given with effective contraception (oestrogen based)
	Cosmetic measures.

CHILDHOOD GYNAECOLOGY

The following list provides an indication of the type of problems encountered:

- congenital abnormalities of the genital tract
- intersex states (abnormal sexual differentiation):
  - female pseudohermaphroditism (female gonads; apparently male external genitalia)
  - male pseudohermaphroditism (male gonads; apparently female external genitalia)
  - true hermaphroditism (very rare)
- trauma to the genital tract
- precocious puberty
- delayed sexual maturation
- tumours, e.g. sarcoma botryoides.

PREMENSTRUAL TENSION SYNDROME

Consists of a symptom complex appearing 1–10 days before the onset of menstruation. Represents an exaggeration of the normal premenstrual phase and is only defined as the premenstrual tension syndrome if it is sufficiently severe to disturb the patient's life. It usually appears when the patient is in her 30s and it has been shown to be an important cause of increased suicide and violent crime amongst women in the premenstrual phase.

Symptoms:

Psychological disturbance:
irritability
moodiness and weepiness
feeling of tension
depression

Fluid retention:
bloated abdomen
tense tender breasts
'sausage fingers'

Miscellaneous:
headaches and migraines
faints
backache
easy bruising.

Treatment:

Suppression of ovulation (with which it is associated) by use of the oral contraceptive pill
Progesterone/progestogen therapy in 2nd half of cycle
Diuretics
Avoid tranquillisers and anti-depressants — psychiatric referral should be arranged if indicated
Mefanamic acid
Supportive counselling
In the 40s consider HRT before cyclical progestogens.

Infertility

Infertility and its investigation, management and treatment is complex but logical and therefore amenable to understanding(!). In basic terms (which can provide the framework for an essay plan) there must be:

- a sperm
- an ovum
- the opportunity for them to get together.

Definitions and statistics

Infertility:

The failure to conceive after 12 to 18 months of regular intercourse without contraception. Subfertility is synonymous. Approximately 1 in 10 couples are affected.

It may be either *primary*, in which the woman has never conceived, or *secondary*, in which there is failure to conceive despite one or more successful or unsuccessful pregnancies in the past.

Sterility:

Means that there is no ability to conceive.

In about 35% of infertile couples, the male is at fault

In about 30% of infertile couples, the female is at fault

In the remainder, both are at fault

In the presence of normal coital activity:

42% of menstrual cycles result in no conception

42% of menstrual cycles result in normal fertilised ova

16% of menstrual cycle result in an ova which will abort

If a woman misses a period, there is approximately a 70% chance of a normal pregnancy, and a 30% chance of a miscarriage.

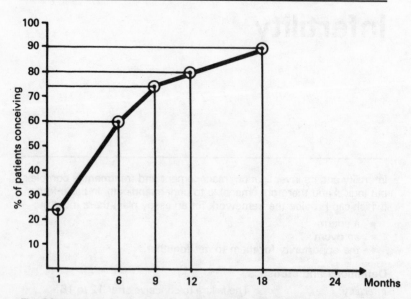

Fig. 20 The percentage of women who conceive after regular unprotected intercourse increases with time. Note that by 18 months 90% will have conceived.

Thorough work-up will identify the cause in 90% of couples. Appropriate treatment will lead to pregnancy in about 40% of couples treated.

A proportion of 'infertile' women will conceive following the first consultation with no treatment once they have 'off-loaded' their problem onto the medical practitioner.

Causes

Female
General: Timing of intercourse
                Frequency of intercourse
                Activities after intercourse:
                    getting up to micturate or douche.

Anatomical:
Congenital: Uterine absence
                Uterine hypoplasia
                Gonadal dysgenesis.

Acquired:	Tubal occlusion at any portion of the tube by:
	  gonorrhoea
	  chlamydia
	  tuberculosis
	Appendicitis and pelvic abscess
	Pelvic adhesions after surgery
	Pelvic adhesions after ectopic pregnancy
	Abnormalities due to endometriosis
	Ashermann's syndrome
	Fibroids, especially submucous fibroids which act like IUCDs
	Cervical and vaginal infections, by making the local environment hostile to sperms
	Iatrogenic: tubal ligation.

Endocrine:	Premature ovarian failure Pituitary failure Raised prolactin due to an adenoma or micro-adenomata Thyroid disorder Adrenal disorder Polycystic ovary syndrome with raised serum testosterone Obesity Anorexia nervosa (some authorities believe that amenorrhoea occurs below a weight of about 7 stone); recent weight loss is important Diabetes mellitus.

Male
Oligospermia means that there is a reduced number of sperms in the ejaculate. Azoospermia means that there are no sperms.

Causes of oligospermia/ azoospermia:	Mumps orchitis Diabetes mellitus Alcohol Smoking Herniorrhaphy — especially in infancy Operations for non-descent/maldescent of the testis Exposure to radiation Chemotheraphy Drugs — Salazopyrin, Dapsone and many others

Toxic substances — lead, copper
Tight underpants
Varicocoele
Hydrocoele
Cryptorchids (remember that an ectopic
  testis can undergo malignant change).

Normal semen analysis suggests possible psychosexual problems, e.g. impotence, premature ejaculation, inability to ejaculate.

Retrograde ejaculation   Bladder neck surgery
caused by: Prostatectomy.

Post-coital MSU in retrograde ejaculation contains sperms.

Normal semen analysis   Volume 2—6 ml
values: Viscosity Full liquefaction in 60 min
                             Sperm density 40–250 $\times$ 10^6/ml
                             Motility 60%
                             Vitality 35% dead
                             Morphology 60% normal.

Remember: 4 ml with more than 40 million/ml with
                             40% abnormal forms and 40% dead.

Sperm counts less than 10^6 per ml or 25 $\times$ 10^6 per ejaculate are uncommon in fertile males.
   3–5% of men show evidence of auto-immunity with circulating antibodies to their own sperms.
   Antibodies may be:

• auto-agglutinating
• auto-immobilising.

Auto-agglutinating antibodies cause clumping of sperm on semen analysis.
Auto-immobilising antibodies cause poor mobility on semen analysis.

Auto-immunity may be   Obstruction to the vas deferens (and may
caused by: therefore be present after reversal of
                             male sterilisation)
                           Inflammatory prostatitis
                           Orchitis
                           Testicular biopsy.

The presence of auto-antibodies may reduce the pregnancy rate by 50% or more.

INVESTIGATION

Diagnosis = History + Examination + Special Tests

A scheme for the investigation of the infertile couple is described below using flow charts. As a useful exercise, the student might like to join the separate flow charts together to clarify how they interrelate. Figure 21 shows an example of a questionnaire to be completed for subfertility patients.

Ideally the couple are seen together.

More realistically, the woman is seen as near to mid-cycle as possible, having had intercourse within the previous 12 hours, this for the purpose of performing a post- coital test.

Points to highlight in the history:

Coital history
Acquired anatomical changes
Contraceptive history
Obstetric history
Drug ingestion
Alcohol consumption (male partner)
Menstrual history
Galactorrhoea (suggests raised prolactin).

On examination look especially for:

Thyroid enlargement/disorder
Galactorrhoea
Physique — hirsutes
Genitalia — abnormality
Cervical and vaginal inflammation and
    discharge (take a smear if not done
    within the past 2 years)
Take bacteriological swabs if indicated
Assess stringiness of cervical mucous
    (Spinnbarkheit)
Aspirate from the endocervix for the
    post-coital test
On bimanual pelvic examination look for:
        uterine abnormality
        thickening of the tubes
        adnexal masses
        thickening of the utero-sacral
        ligaments
        tenderness.

Special Tests:

FBC ESR
VD Serology
Rubella titres (so that you don't have to
    worry about contacts if treatment is
    successful)

FERTILITY QUESTIONNAIRE

FEMALE PART

Date:
Age:
Race:
Work:
Years Married:
Previous Marriage: STERILE   FERTILE
Years Tried:
Family History:

Illnesses: TB RF DM Jaundice
GC Syphilis
Appendicectomy
Lower Abdominal Ops.
Renal Tract Infection
Allergies
Other Illness
Other Ops.

Drugs:
Alcohol:
Smoking:
Previous Fertility Investigations:

Intercourse: Frequency
Timing
Gets Up After Intercourse?
Orgasm
Dyspareunia
Frigidity
Vaginal Lubricants
Previous Pregnancies: LIVEBIRTH STILLBIRTH

Miscarriages (present or previous partnership):
Sterility: PRIMARY SECONDARY

Contraception: Pill
Sheath
Cap
Chemical
Withdrawal
IUCD

Gynaecological History:
LMP:
Menarche
K = / ; Heavy/Light
Pain/No pain
IMB
PCB
PMT
Dyspareunia: Deep/Superficial
Mittelschmerz
Vaginal Discharge
Breasts: Lumps Nipple Discharge
Bowels
Bladder
Height
Weight: Recent Loss?
Recent Smear?
Rubella Immunisation?   BCG?

MALE PART

Name
Age
Work
Children?
Illnesses: Mumps
Orchitis
GC
Syphilis
Hernia
Hernia Op.
Testes
TB RF DM Jaundice
Other Ops.:
Alcohol:
Drugs:
Intercourse:
Impotence
Penetration
Premature Ejac.
Other coital problems:

Fig. 21 Suggested questionnaire for subfertility patients

FBC; ESR
21-day progesterone
Serum prolactin
Chest X-ray if TB salpingitis a possibility
If amenorrhoeic/oligomenorrhoeic do TFTs
    FSH + LH
Endometrial biopsy, specimens being
    sent for TB culture as well as
    histopathology. Such biopsies may be
    taken later at the time of laparoscopy,
    ideally in the premenstrual phase. The
    non-invasive investigations should be
    completed first.
Hysteroscopy at time of laparoscopy.
Endocervical swab

By now we should be able to start sorting out infertile couples into
different groups like this:

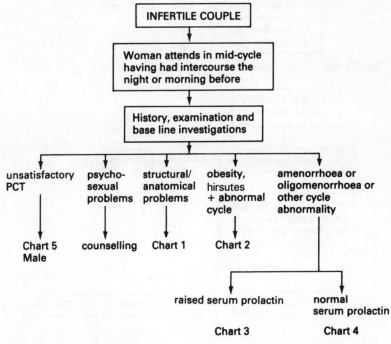

Fig. 22 Guide to flow charts

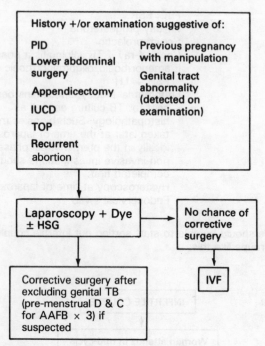

Fig. 23 Flow chart 1: Structural/anatomical problems

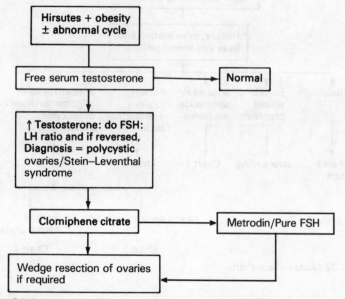

Fig. 24 Flow chart 2: Hirsutes + obesity + abnormal cycle

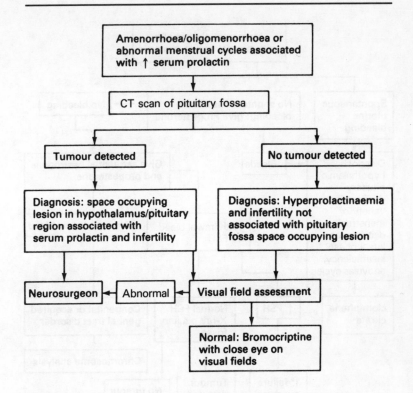

Fig. 25 Flow chart 3: Menstrual abnormalities associated with ↑ serum prolactin

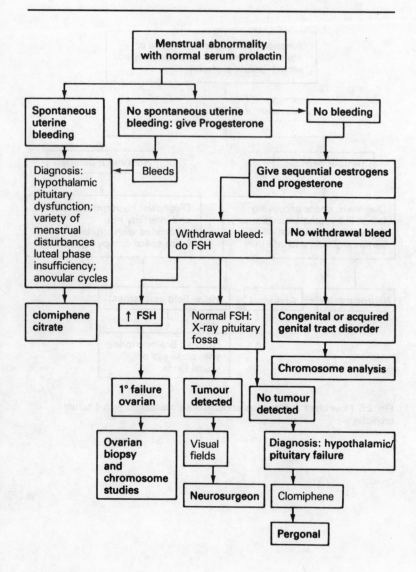

Fig. 26 Flow chart 4: Menstrual abnormality associated with normal serum prolactin

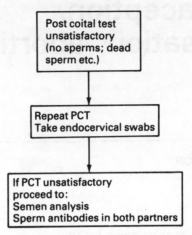

Fig. 27 Flow chart 5

By this stage, a full work-up on the male partner should have been undertaken.

Further investigation should include cross-hostility testing of the sperm and cervical mucus.

Electron microscopy of sperm, especially the tail is now being performed.

Management

Low sperm count (oligospermia)
Check medication
Stop alcohol abuse
Wear loose underpants
Bathe testicles in cold water
Correct hydrocoele, varicocoele
Try giving zinc sulphate
Try clomiphene citrate
Try gonadotrophins
Artificial insemination by husband using split ejaculate. (Most sperms
    are in the first part of the ejaculate.)

No sperms (azoospermia)
If this is iatrogenic due to vasectomy then reversal may be attempted. Plastic urological procedures may be attempted on the bladder neck if there is retrograde ejaculation.

Artificial insemination by donor.

Finally, if there is no chance of the couple conceiving, they should be counselled about adoption and the several adoption agencies.

Contraception, sterilisation, abortion

CONTRACEPTION

Traditional
Chemical
Mechanical
Hormonal
Intra-uterine contraceptive device (IUCD)
Sterilisation.

Pearl Index
Measure of effectiveness of contraceptive.

$$PI = \frac{\text{Total Accidental Pregnancies}}{\text{Total Months of Contraceptive Exposure}} \times 1200$$

= Number of pregnancies/100 years of contraceptive exposure i.e. the lower the PI, the better the contraceptive.

Traditional

Male:	Coitus interruptus	(PI = 10–38)
	Coitus saxonicus (pressure on urethra to divert ejaculate into bladder)	
Female:	Lactation (prolongation of)	(PI = 24–26)
	Rhythm (safe period)	(PI = 24–38)

Chemical
Vaginal douche (PI = 21–41)
Spermicidal foam, jelly, cream, (PI = 4–43)
'C-film' (may also mechanically
  inhibit sperm and provide
  prophylaxis against STD).

Side-effects:
Sensitisation to agents used (either partner).

Mechanical

Male:	Condom	(PI = 7–28)
	(Also provides prophylaxis against STD including HIV) Effectiveness very dependent on how used.	

Female:	Diaphragm (Dutch cap)	(PI = 4–35)
	Cervical caps Both should be used with spermicidal cream Effectiveness very dependent on how used. Female condom	

Hormonal
Combined pill (high or low oestrogen)   (PI = 0.03–0.1)
Progestogen-only (mini-pill)   (PI = 2–7)
Correct pill taking essential to achieve
contraception
Depot (parenteral) progestogens

Oestrogen → Inhibits FSH → Inhibits ovulation.

Mechanism of action
  (i) Oestrogen component inhibits ovulation by inhibiting FSH production by the anterior pituitary
 (ii) Inhibits LH releasing factor production
(iii) Progestogen component keeps cervical mucous viscid to the detriment of sperm transport, and produces hostile changes in the endometrium.
     Progestogen-only pills are taken daily at the same time.

Contraindications to combined pill
Pregnancy
DVT and thrombo-embolic disorders
Liver disease and recurrent jaundice
Breast and uterine cancer
Sickle cell disease
Hyperlipidaemia.

Be cautious about use in:
Diabetes mellitus
Hypertension
Patients over 35 years who smoke (progestogen-only pill OK)
The obese

Lactating mothers
Epilepsy
Cardiac and renal disease.

Side-effects
Oestrogen
- Weight gain, fluid retention
- Nausea, vomiting
- Headache
- Hypertension
  Impairment of liver function
  Benign hepatic tumours
  Reduced venous flow in legs
  Increase in size of fibroids.

Progestogen
- Breast tenderness
- Acne
  Depression
- Headache
- Hirsutism
- Loss of libido
  Weight gain (steady)
  Dry vagina
  Reduced menstrual loss
  Cervical erosion.

Drug interactions reducing the effect of oral contraceptives
Antibiotics
Barbiturates
Carbamazepine
Phenytoin
Rifampicin
(Gastrointestinal disturbance).

Oral contraceptives reduce the effect of:
Antihypertensive drugs
Diuretics
Warfarin
Phenindione
Tricyclic antidepressants
Oral hypoglycaemics
Insulin.

Injectable contraceptives
Medroxyprogesterone acetate (a progestogen)
   (PI = 0.5–1.5).

Useful for short-term contraception:
    (1) after vasectomy
    (2) rubella immunisation.
Use may be followed by transient infertility and irregular cycles.
Now approved for long-term contraception.
Useful for those who have difficulty remembering to take the pill
and/or have infrequent intercourse.

Missed pill guidelines
(Applies only to combined pills)

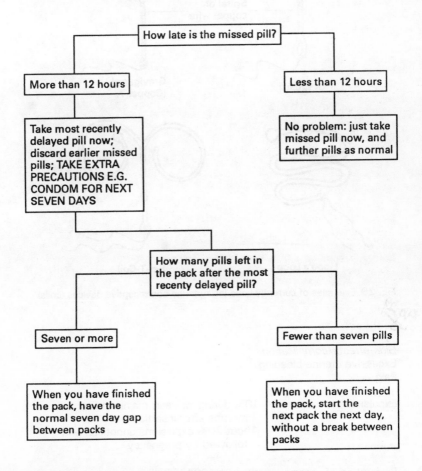

Fig. 28 Guidelines on missed combined contraceptive pills

Intra-uterine contraceptive devices (IUCDs)

Pearl Index (overall for different types) 0.8–5.8.

New copper bearing devices (such as Novaguard) may be left in for 5 years.

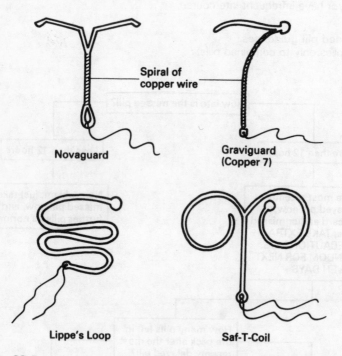

Spiral of
copper wire

Novaguard

**Graviguard
(Copper 7)**

Lippe's Loop

Saf-T-Coil

Fig. 29 Examples of currently used intra-uterine contraceptive devices (coils)

Side-effects/complications
Excessive uterine bleeding
Pain

Expulsion: 10% during lst year; mainly in first few
                      months after insertion
                      About 20% expulsions unnoticed and
                      followed by pregnancy

Perforation of uterus: about 1:1000 insertions.

Device detected by:	X-ray: AP and lateral of pelvis AP and lateral of abdomen Ultrasound scan may help Contrast in uterus may help (sound or dye).
Pelvic inflammatory disease:	<30 days after insertion — probably due to IUCD <30 days after insertion — probably venereal in origin Coil may left in for initial treatment of infection.

1:20 chance of ectopic pregnancy if become pregnant with IUCD in situ.

If intra-uterine pregnancy plus coil:	Gentle attempt at removal with patient's informed consent If coil is stuck, leave in situ 50% chance of abortion No effect on fetus.

Sterilisation

Male:	Vasectomy.
Female:	Tubal occlusion.
Pre-operative considerations:	Age (most women requesting reversal of sterilisation were sterilised below the age of 30) Marital stability Medical fitness Counselling Previous abdominal/pelvic surgery.
Vasectomy:	Safe Simple Usually done under local anaesthesia 1 cm segment of vas deferens removed Not immediately effective: absence of sperm must be confirmed in two ejaculates, 1 month apart.

Tubal occlusion

Many different methods:	Laparoscopic Laparotomy.

Laparoscopic: Falope rings (tiny elastic bands)
                       Clips
                       Diathermy coagulation.

Laparotomy: Fimbriectomy
                       Salpingectomy (bilateral)
                       Pomeroy tubal ligation
                       Hysterectomy.

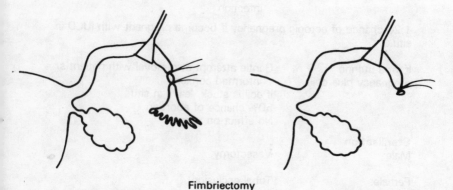

Fimbriectomy

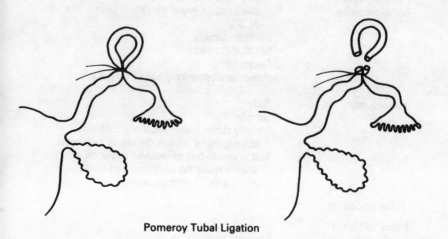

Pomeroy Tubal Ligation

Fig. 30 Two methods of female sterilisation

Although each method is intended to be irreversible, permanence cannot be guaranteed, with the exception of bilateral salpingectomy and hysterectomy.

Counselling pre-operatively should stress these points and inform patient that failure of sterilisation could result in a tubal ectopic pregnancy.

Complications
Hazards of any anaesthetic
Hazards of any operation
Diathermy coagulation: risk of thermal damage to other structures
Psychological/psychiatric sequelae
Failure, e.g. due to ligation of round ligament by mistake.

Side-effects
Approximately 20–40% of women subsequently undergo hysterectomy for menstrual problems.

Induced abortion
Considered for medical or non-medical reasons.

Medical reasons: Fetal abnormality
                              Blighted ovum/missed abortion
                              Renal disease
                              Certain cardiac disorders
                              Recurrent severe pre-eclampsia
                              Previous vesico-vaginal fistula repair
                              Pulmonary TB
                              Leukaemia
                              Psychiatric disorder.

Recently the Abortion Act has been amended to take into account the fact that a fetus of 24 weeks' gestation is viable. See new Certificate A (Fig. 31).
Majority performed under clause C.

IN CONFIDENCE

CERTIFICATE A

ABORTION ACT 1967

Not to be destroyed within three years of the date of operation

Certificate to be completed before an abortion is
performed under Section 1(1) of the Act

I, ...

(Name and qualifications of practitioner in block capitals)

of ....

....

(Full address of practitioner)

Have/have not* seen/and examined* the pregnant woman to whom this certificate relates at

....

....

(full address of place at which patient was seen or examined)

on ....

and I ....

(Name and qualifications of practitioner in block capitals)

of ....

....

(Full address of practitioner)

Have/have not* seen/and examined* the pregnant woman to whom this certificate relates at

....

....

(Full address of place at which patient was seen or examined)

on ....

We hereby certify that we are of the opinion, formed in good faith, that in the case

of ....

(Full name of pregnant woman in block capitals)

of ....

....

(Usual place of residence of pregnant woman in block capitals)

(Ring appropriate letter(s))	A	the continuance of the pregnancy would involve risk to the life of the pregnant woman greater than if the pregnancy were terminated;
	B	the termination is necessary to prevent grave permanent injury to the physical or mental health of the pregnant woman;
	C	the pregnancy has NOT exceeded its 24th week and that the continuance of the pregnancy would involve risk, greater than if the pregnancy were terminated, of injury to the physical or mental health of the pregnant woman;
	D	the pregnancy has NOT exceeded its 24th week and that the continuance of the pregnancy would involve risk, greater than if the pregnancy were terminated, of injury to the physical or mental health of any existing child(ren) of the family of the pregnant woman;
	E	there is a substantial risk that if the child were born it would suffer from such physical or mental abnormalities as to be seriously handicapped.

This certificate of opinion is given before the commencement of the treatment for the termination of pregnancy to which it refers and relates to the circumstances of the pregnant woman's individual case.

Signed ....   Date ....

Signed ....   Date ....

* Delete as appropriate   Printed in the U.K. for H.M.S.O 2/91 Dd.DH000759 C10000 38806 G3759   Form HSA1 (revised 1991)

Fig. 31 Certificate A (1992). (Crown copyright. Reproduced with permission of the Controller of Her Majesty's Stationery Office.)

Methods

Vacuum aspiration: 1st trimester (occasionally up to 16 weeks' gestation).

NB All vaginal suction terminations risk cervical damage and subsequent mid- trimester abortion.

Mid-trimester

Extra– or intra-amniotic prostaglandins

Intra-amniotic urea

Hysterotomy and hysterectomy (unusual in modern practice).

Complications of early pregnancy

ABORTION

Definition: Termination of pregnancy (spontaneous or induced) before 24 weeks' duration. It should be remembered that whilst the terms miscarriage and abortion may be medically synonymous, for patients they are often not.

A fetus lost after 24 weeks' gestation must be registered as a still-birth, and a Still Birth Certificate issued. This is because a fetus of 24 weeks' gestation or more is considered to be viable.

Incidence: Very common: quoted rates vary between 1 in every 2 conceptions to 1 in every 10, the difficulty being in recognising the event. A useful day to day figure is 1 in 3. The incidence decreases as the pregnancy advances, e.g. 1:2 below 12 weeks; 1:200 at 16 weeks.

Abortion is an extremely important subject, not least because it represents a major source of maternal morbidity and mortality.

Classification: Spontaneous abortion (as opposed to induced abortion, see p. 109) may be viewed as a process which passes through identifiable stages. This progression provides a classification based on which stage has been reached:
Threatened
Inevitable
Incomplete
Complete
or
Missed.

Additional
classification is by:

Time:
   early 0–12 weeks
   late (mid-trimester) 12–28 weeks
Infection present or absent:
   septic
   non-septic
Frequency of occurrence:
   habitual recurrent abortion
   — three consecutive abortions

Clinical features of abortion

Abortion may present at any of the stages listed above.

Threatened abortion

Definition:

Any uterine bleeding in a woman with an intra-uterine pregnancy of less than 24 weeks' completed gestation occurring in the absence of cervical dilatation, ± pain.

The extragenital features of pregnancy (delayed menstruation, breast tenderness, etc.) are usually present.

The blood may be red or brown, and the volume of blood lost varies.

Backache may be present but pain is usually not a feature: its presence suggests progression to the next stage — inevitable abortion.

Inevitable abortion

Definition:

Inevitable abortion occurs when threatened abortion progresses to the stage of cervical dilatation. Loss of the pregnancy is now 'inevitable'.

Progression from threatened to inevitable abortion is often indicated by cramping lower abdominal pain. (Sacral pain strongly suggests cervical dilatation.)

Bleeding is usually more profuse.

Incomplete abortion

Definition:

Incomplete abortion occurs when abortion progresses to the point when some but not all of the products of conception have been expelled from the uterus.

Pain ('cramps' as the uterus tries to expel the residual products) and bleeding (because the uterus is unable to contract adequately because of the residual products) are usually present. Bleeding may be very severe leading to shock, and require urgent removal of products from the cervical os with sponge holders in A and E.

Complete abortion

Definition: Complete abortion has occurred when the uterus has expelled all the products of conception. Pain stops and bleeding stops or is greatly reduced.

Missed abortion

Definition: Fetal death in utero without its expulsion prior to 28 weeks' gestation. Although not strictly part of the process of abortion, it is often considered with it.
  Presents with failure of progression of the pregnancy: cessation of uterine enlargement, and regression of the clinical features of pregnancy. May be found at booking clinic, completely unexpected by mother — tact is needed.

Diagnosis: Negative pregnancy test following previously positive test, although may remain positive. Ultrasound: no fetal heart movements, or an anembryonic pregnancy.

Management: Evacuation of the uterus as soon as practicable, usually by suction, but occasionally by inducing a miscarriage with prostaglandins
Prophylactic antibiotics post ERPC are wise.

Complications: Sepsis
Disseminated intravascular coagulation
Psychological disturbance of mother.

Recurrent (habitual) abortion

Definition: Three or more consecutive abortions which may be early or mid-trimester. The implication is that the abortions are due to recurrent factors rather than accidental causes and therefore investigation and treatment where possible is appropriate.

Causes: Any cause of abortion but in particular:
parental chromosome abnormality
maternal uterine abnormality
chronic maternal ill health (e.g. diabetes, renal failure)
incompetent cervix (usually causes mid-trimester abortion, q.v.)
maternal infection — CMV, rubella, toxoplasmosis, brucellosis.
in practice, a cause is often not found in recurrent 1st trimester abortion (cf. mid-trimester abortion).

Investigation: Chromosome analysis
Hysterosalpingogram and cervicogram
WR, CXR, urinalysis (i.e. screening general health of the patient)
Thyroid function tests (come in and out of vogue)
Rubella, CMV, toxoplasma, herpes titres, (TORCH screen: now considered to be of little value
Listeria titres — again of little value.

Treatment: Apart from correction of specific identifiable causes, *no treatment has been proven to prevent recurrent early abortion.*
The following have been tried:
progesterone supplements (not those based on testosterone)
specific attention to diet and vitamins (especially folic acid and vitamin C pre-conception)
rest and correction of anaemia
avoiding intercourse at times of greatest risk
white cell immunotherapy
junior aspirin
treatment of autoimmune condition.

Mid-trimester (late) abortion
In contrast to 1st trimester abortion, mid-trimester abortion is less common, but more often recurrent when it does occur, and a cause is usually identifiable. Investigation after the first loss is therefore appropriate.

Causes:	Incompetent cervix (recognised by painless abortion — the fetus 'drops out' and often a history of previous gynaecological surgery involving cervical trauma is present) Maternal uterine abnormality Fetal abnormality and intra-uterine death (the expelled fetus should be sent for laboratory examination if possible) High order multiple pregnancy and/or hydramnios Maternal ill health UTI (may be silent).
Treatment:	Shirodkar (or similar) suture for incompetent cervix (less frequently performed — doubt as to usefulness) Surgical correction of uterine abnormality Treatment of maternal ill health as appropriate Regular screening for UTI ± treatment.

General causes of abortion
Patients (and examiners) often wish to know why abortion occurs. Often in a particular case the cause is not known, but the following provides a list of possible causes. Special considerations apply to mid-trimester abortion.

Fetal causes (most common and not recurrent):	Gross malformation Chromosome abnormality Failure of implantation.
Maternal causes:	Corpus luteum insufficiency Uterine abnormalities Cervical incompetence Maternal ill health/infection.
Mutual factors:	Failure of immune tolerance.

In day to day practice abortion without obvious cause is usually assumed to be due to fetal abnormality. Some patients may appreciate the idea that when there is fetal abnormality, abortion represents nature's way of getting rid of 'bad' fetuses.

Management of abortion

Diagnosis:

The history and general examination will suggest the diagnosis

Opinions vary concerning the advisability of vaginal examination; usually gentle examination is acceptable to the patient (and most consultants) and allows differentiation between threatened and inevitable abortion

Ultrasound scan

Pregnancy test.

Treatment:

The treatment depends on the stage:

Threatened abortion: 1 in 3 will progress to inevitable abortion and it is doubtful whether any therapy alters the outcome; however, any or all of the following may be used:

bed rest

sedation, especially for active patients for whom bed rest is difficult

avoidance of intercourse

progesterone supplements

reassurance to the mother that if the pregnancy does continue the fetus is likely to be normal.

Inevitable and incomplete abortion:

General measures including treatment of shock and/or infection if present.

If required, urgent control of haemorrhage may be attempted by removal of products or with ergometrine 0.5 mg i.m./i.v.

The definitive treatment is surgical (evacuation of the uterus — ERPC (evacuation of retained products of conception).

Complete abortion:

Accurately diagnosed, requires no treatment

If in doubt, best to perform ERPC
(Ultrasound scan may be used to exclude
the presence of retained products —
however, often useful to 'document'
pregnancy with histopathology of
products of conception)
Don't forget psychological issues.

ECTOPIC PREGNANCY

Definition: Pregnancy in which implantation of the
fertilised ovum occurs outside the uterine
cavity.

Incidence: 0.3% of normal births (not pregnancies)
5–10% recurrence rate (in addition to
which a woman has only 1 in 3 chance of
a normal pregnancy after an ectopic
pregnancy).

Mortality: Ectopic pregnancy accounts for 9% of
maternal mortality, (1985–1987).

Risk factors: Previous ectopic pregnancy
Pelvic inflammatory disease (especially due
    to gonococcus and tuberculosis)
Tubal surgery
Intra-uterine contraceptive device per se
    (not as a result of infection caused by
    the device) but note that this is a relative
    increase only: the absolute rate is
    decreased since the device is itself a
    contraceptive
Increased incidence in negroes
Progestogen-only pills (see note about
    relative and absolute rates above).

Sites of implantation: Ampulla of tube ⎫ tubal pregnancy
Isthmus of tube ⎬ (95% of all ectopic
                 ⎭ pregnancies)
Ovary: rare
Abdomen: rare
Cervix: very rare.

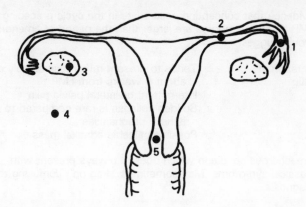

Fig. 32 Sites of implantation in ectopic pregnancy: (1) ampulla of tube; (2) isthmus of tube; (3)ovary; (4) abdominal cavity; (5) cervix

Pathophysiology/ outcome:	Depends on site:
	   isthmus of tube — tubal rupture
	   ampulla of tube — tubal rupture or
	     abortion (extrusion via end of tube)
	   ovary — usually ruptures
	   abdomen — may proceed to term —
	     rare.

Clinical features:	Clinical features of early pregnancy:
	   delayed menstruation
	   breast changes
	   early morning sickness
	   frequency of micturition
	Postural hypotension
	Further features depend on the site:

Implantation at isthmus:	Tends to present 'acutely' at about 4–6
	   weeks from LMP
	Severe lower abdominal ± shoulder tip
	   (referred diaphragmatic) pain
	Dark vaginal blood loss, typically after the
	   pain — 'prune juice' vaginal loss
	Shock and signs of peritonism.
	Vaginal tenderness with marked cervical
	   excitation on vaginal examination (which
	   should only be done in hospital
	   because of the risk of provoking further
	   bleeding).

NB Evidence that conception occurs late in the cycle preceding the
   LMP as most embryos are larger than the period of amenorrhoea
   would suggest.

Implantation at   Tends to present rather less acutely at
ampulla: about 6 weeks from LMP
                               Intermittent unilateral pelvic pain
                               Sudden collapse is rare compared to
                                  isthmal pregnancies.
                               Possible palpable adnexal mass.

NB Treacherous condition which doesn't always present with
   classical symptoms. May sometimes 'drag on', confusing the
   diagnosis.

Differential diagnosis: Only common diagnoses are listed:
                                  appendicitis
                                  pelvic inflammatory disease
                                  ruptured corpus luteum cyst/ovarian cyst
                                  uterine abortion
                                  urinary tract infection.

Management of ectopic pregnancy
The management depends on the gravity of the situation.
Seriously ill, shocked patient with 'certain' diagnosis:
   Resuscitation = IVI with blood, continue and perform laparotomy
   as soon as possible. Usual definitive procedure:
   salpingectomy.
Probable ectopic pregnancy, but patient not gravely ill:
   Diagnostic EUA ± laparoscopy followed by laparotomy and
   salpingectomy if required.
Patient in whom the diagnosis only a possibility:
   Ultrasound scan of pelvis: note intra-uterine pregnancy does not
   exclude co-existent ectopic pregnancy: ectopic pregnancy must be
   specifically looked for. In practice, an ultrasound may confirm an
   ectopic but can rarely exclude one.
   βHCG pregnancy test kits allow the detection of early pregnancy.
   Vaginal examination is essential. At the end of the day, laparoscopy
   remains the cornerstone for investigating suspected ectopics. If
   pain persists for more than 24 hours despite a negative βHCG
   pregnancy test, laparascopy should be done.
   Curettage of the uterus (for whatever reason) may produce
   intra-uterine decidua but no chorionic tissue, or the Arias Stella
   phenomenon may be seen. These two findings suggest the
   presence of an ectopic pregnancy.

NB Conservative surgery for ectopic becoming more common i.e.,
   tube segment + ectopic resected only.

TROPHOBLASTIC DISEASE

Rare but important spectrum of 'diseases' ranging from normal
trophoblast tissue (which itself is capable of invasion and metastasis)
to choriocarcinoma. The spectrum includes:

- Normal 'metastatic' trophoblast (e.g. in the lungs)
- Hydatidiform mole
- Invasive mole
- Choriocarcinoma.

The matter is further confused by the fact that one manifestation of
the disease may progress to or arise from another manifestation of
the disease (see Fig. 30 below). Additional discussion of the disease
is on pp. 66–67.

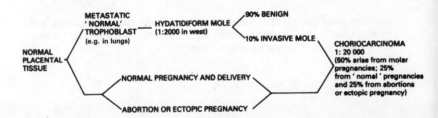

Fig. 33 Trophoblastic disease: inter relations and rates of incidence

MINIMALLY INVASIVE SURGERY

In gynaecology:

- laparoscopy
- hysteroscopy
- the procedures that can be performed via these routes.

Laparoscopy: Diagnostic, for pain
Dye tests of fallopian tube patency
Division of peri-tubal and ovarian adhesions
Aspiration of ovarian cysts
Laser or cautery to pelvic endometriosis
Salpingotomy and evacuation of ectopic
  pregnancy
Salpingectomy
Oöphorectomy
Gamete intra-fallopian transfer (sub-fertile
  women with patent tubes).

(Some surgeons are now advocating laparoscopic hysterectomy, a dubious procedure in view of the ease with which vaginal hysterectomy can be performed.)

Hysteroscopy: Diagnostic with endometrial biopsy
Trans-cervical resection of the endometrium (for menorrhagia)
Resection of polyps and sub-mucous fibroids
Division of adhesions within uterine cavity
Contact hysteroscopy can be used to diagnose early neoplasia
Tuboscopy can be performed and the tubes cannulated.

As time goes on, more indications for minimally invasive surgery will be recognised. It is important that such developments should be in the patient's best interests and be logical.

Obstetrics

PART 3

Obstetrics

Antenatal care. 1: Normal

NORMAL PHYSIOLOGY

Many physiological reference values are changed in pregnancy and therefore it is necessary to know the nature of these changes in order to be able to interpret values determined during pregnancy.

Endocrine changes during pregnancy
See also pp. 16–18 which contain additional information on endocrinology.

Oestrogens (including oestradiol, oestriol)
Oestrogen levels rise progressively in maternal plasma during pregnancy, this rise being reflected in urinary oestrogen secretion (see Fig. 34).

Serial assay of oestriol (which is produced mainly by the fetus) can be used clinically to monitor fetal well-being, especially in late pregnancy (going out of fashion).

Progesterone
As its name suggests, represents the main pro-gestational hormone. Overall levels rise during pregnancy as shown in Figure 35.

Human chorionic gonadotrophin (HCG)
Levels rise rapidly in early pregnancy both in maternal plasma and urine and as such provide a useful basis for a pregnancy test.

Levels plateau after 10–12 weeks and do not change much thereafter (see Fig. 36).

Human placental lactogen (HPL)
Produced by the placenta in progressively larger quantities as the pregnancy proceeds: (see Fig. 37).

May be used clinically as a placental function test (going out of use).

125

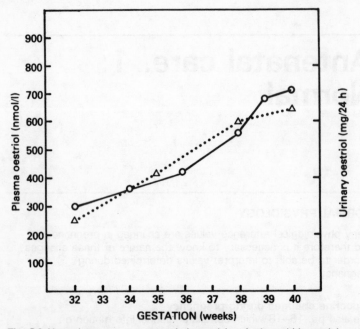

Fig. 34 Normal pregnancy: maternal plasma (o) and urinary (△) oestriol concentration during the last trimester; the rise shown may be absent if there is fetal pathology

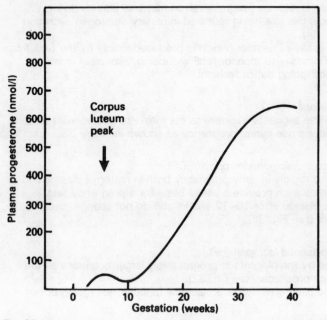

Fig. 35 Normal pregnancy: maternal plasma progesterone concentration

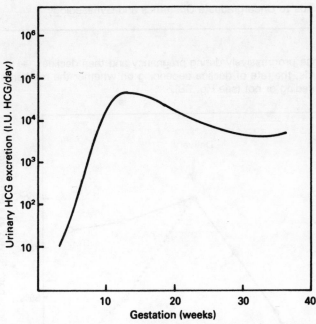

Fig. 36 Normal pregnancy: maternal urinary HCG excretion (note log-linear plot)

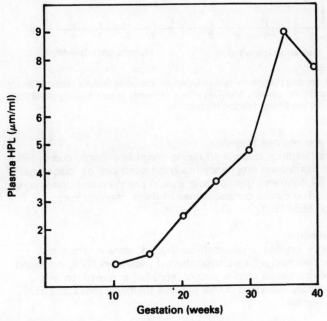

Fig. 37 Normal pregnancy: maternal plasma HPL concentration

Prolactin

Levels rise progressively during pregnancy and then decline afterwards, the rate of decline depending on whether the mother is breast feeding or not (see Fig. 38).

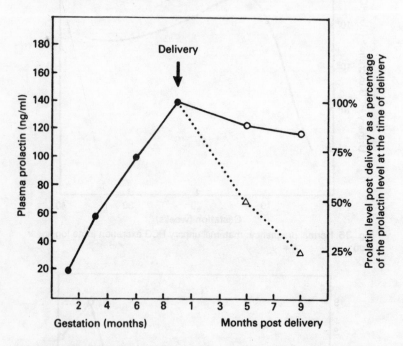

Fig. 38 Normal pregnancy and puerperium: maternal plasma prolactin levels before and after delivery showing effect of mainly breast feeding (solid line) and mainly not breast feeding (dotted line)

Insulin and glucose tolerance

Glucose tolerance is impaired during pregnancy (partly due to HPL) and for this reason pregnancy has been described as 'diabetogenic'. Figure 39 illustrates glucose tolerance in pregnant and non-pregnant women. The clinical consequences of these changes vary (see pp. 165–167).

Thyroid status

Pregnancy induces a 'pseudohyperthyroid' state in which the pregnant women appears hyperthyroid (increased BMR, increased total T4, increased cardiac output, etc.) but in reality remains biochemically euthyroid in that her free thyroxine index and TSH remain normal.

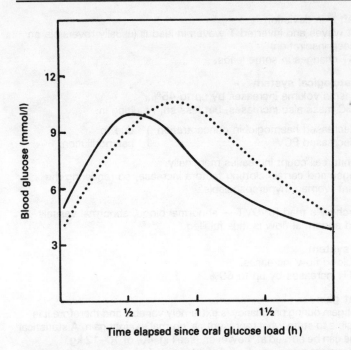

Fig. 39 Glucose tolerance curves in pregnant (dotted line) and non- pregnant women (solid line)

Adrenal function
Glucocorticoid and mineralocorticoid secretion are both increased in pregnancy.

Cardiovascular system
Cardiac output increases by approximately 30% in the first trimester, and then remains reasonably constant until term. Most of the increased output goes to the:

- uterus
- kidneys
- skin.

Blood pressure changes relatively little.
Peripheral resistance drops; venous pressure increases in the lower limbs (pelvic mass effect) but not elsewhere; veins dilate (hence tendency for pregnancy to cause varicose veins).
The ECG becomes modified, mainly as a result of the heart being pushed upwards and laterally by the growing uterus, commonly resulting in:

- left axis deviation
- Q waves and inverted T waves in lead III (usually reversible on deep inspiration)
- ST changes in some leads.

Haematological system
The plasma volume increases by up to 45%.
The RBC mass also increases, but less so, resulting in:

- decreased haemoglobin concentration ⎫ due to
- decreased PCV   ⎬ haemodilution.

The white cell count increases marginally.
Fibrinogen and certain clotting factors increase, so rendering the pregnant woman 'hypercoagulable'.

NB Virchow's triad for DVT — abnormal blood, abnormal vessels and abnormal flow is thus fulfilled.

Renal system
Renal blood flow increases.
The GFR increases by up to 60%.

Weight gain
Weight gain during pregnancy is extremely variable and therefore it is impossible to state what represents a 'normal' weight gain. A statistical average can be arrived at, however, (see Fig. 40) of 10–12 kg.
   Fetal weight gain is more predictable (and of course more important, but less accessible): mean weight gain is shown in Figure 41.

DIAGNOSIS OF PREGNANCY

Relies on the same principles as any other diagnosis:

History: Delayed menstruation
                         Breast fullness and tenderness
                         Urinary tract symptoms, especially
                             frequency
                         Nausea.

Examination: Increased uterine size
                         Cervical softening
                         Increased breast activity, e.g. dilated
                             superficial veins.

Laboratory   Urine HCG assay (the 'standard' pregnancy
investigations: test)
                         Ultrasound scanning
                         β sub-unit HCG (serum) for very early
                             determination of pregnancy.

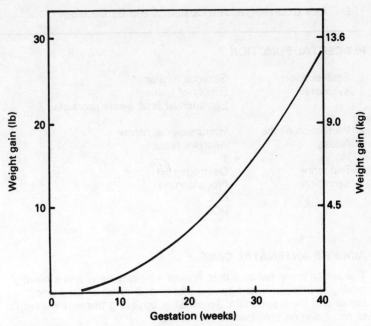

Fig. 40 Mean maternal weight gain during pregnancy

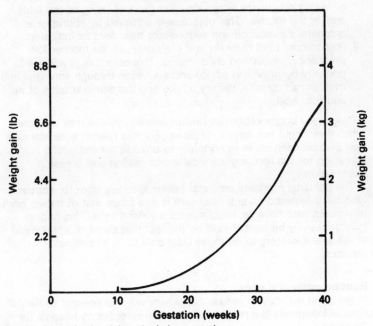

Fig. 41 Mean fetal weight gain during gestation

PLACENTAL FUNCTION

1. Fetal support systems:
   Gaseous exchange
   Supply of nutrients
   Excretion of fetal waste products.

2. Protection of the fetus:
   Immunological barrier
   Anchors fetus.

3. Endocrine secretion:
   Oestrogen
   Progesterone
   HPL
   HCG.

AIMS OF ANTENATAL CARE

The aim of antenatal care is to ensure a healthy baby and a healthy mother, neither of whom have suffered as a result of pregnancy, labour and the puerperium. To assist in achieving this aim it is helpful to recognise certain specific objectives:

1. Prevention, detection and treatment of any disorders arising from or during pregnancy which threaten the well-being of the fetus and/or the mother. This objective is achieved by appropriate antenatal surveillance and subsequent treatment as indicated.
2. Preparation, both mentally and physically, of the mother for pregnancy, labour and child-rearing. This objective is achieved primarily by providing advice and education through antenatal and mothercraft classes, dietary advice and the administration of iron and folic acid.

Pregnancy brings otherwise healthy women to see their doctors when they might not otherwise do so. For this reason antenatal care may also be seen as an opportunity to provide general health screening for women, e.g. cervical smear testing and breast examination.

The perinatal mortality amongst babies who are born to women who have received no antenatal care is five times that of babies born to women who have received normal antenatal care. This finding may, however, be confounded by the fact that those mothers most at risk are also likely to be those least able to 'use' antenatal services.

Routine antenatal care

In the great majority of cases, the patient will first present to her GP who will diagnose the pregnancy and then refer her to hospital for 'booking'.

First hospital visit (booking clinic)
Normally done at about 12–16 weeks.

Attention is focused
on:

Confirming diagnosis of pregnancy
Establishing the dating of the pregnancy
Collecting baseline and background
    information
Identification of risk factors.

History:

This pregnancy
Previous pregnancies
Gynaecological history
Menstrual history
Medical history — including smoking,
    alcohol, drugs
Family and social history
Ethnic group.
(Check out the antenatal notes at your
    hospital and use these as a framework
    for clerking your case in the clinicals).

Examination:

Weight and height
Blood pressure
Urinalysis
Cardiovascular system
Respiratory system
Breasts
Thyroid
Abdomen
(Pelvis [including speculum] not essential)
Teeth
Varicose veins

Investigations:

Haemoglobin plus electrophoresis if
    appropriate
ABO and rhesus blood grouping, with
    antibody screen
VDRL
Rubella antibodies
EMU — ward testing
HVS if appropriate
Ultrasound scan for:
    dating the pregnancy (not obligatory)
    provision of baseline for further growth
    detection of abnormalities, e.g.
        multiple pregnancy
Current practice:
    anomaly scan at 18–20 weeks
    cardiac anomaly scan at about 24 weeks.

Subsequent visits

1. Frequently shared with the general practitioner/midwife.
2. Schedule of visits takes account of the fact that the frequency of complications increases with the duration of the pregnancy:

    monthly until 28 weeks and then ⎫ unless
    fortnightly until 36 weeks and then ⎬ otherwise
    weekly until delivery ⎭ indicated.

3. Focus of attention changes as pregnancy progresses:
    (a) second trimester (usually an 'uneventful' trimester)
        (i) general assessment of fetal growth
        (ii) early detection of maternal complications including pre-eclampsia, anaemia, etc.
    (b) third trimester
        (i) assessment of fetal maturity, growth and well-being
        (ii) maternal well-being
        (iii) mechanics of and/or possible need for intervention in labour.
4. Clinical assessment at each visit:
    (a) weight
    (b) blood pressure
    (c) urinalysis (protein and glucose)
    (d) oedema
    (e) abdomen
        (i) uterine size
        (ii) fetal viability (fetal heart and/or movements)
        (iii) fetal lie
        (iv) fetal presentation
        (v) fetal abnormality (including amount of liquor)
        (vi) engagement of the presenting part
        (vii) abdominal examination for the position of the fetal back is of little value.
5. Additional investigations:
    haemoglobin at 28 and 34 weeks
    rhesus antibodies (if appropriate) at 28 and 34 weeks
    ultrasound scans — BPD and abdominal circumference if IUGR suspected, or if twins or PET
    fetal kick charts
    cardiotocograph monitoring.
    The last three should be done as often as indicated.

ANTENATAL ADVICE FOR MOTHER

Consider under various headings:

1. Diet: Well-balanced
                            Increase protein and calcium intake
                            Routine iron and vitamin supplements.

2. Lifestyle: Stop smoking
                             Stop alcohol consumption
                             Work up until 32 weeks if wanted
                             Moderate amounts of exercise, plenty of
                                 rest
                             Sex — couples' own inclinations are the
                                 best guide unless medical indications
                                 override.

3. Dental care: Gingivitis very common in pregnancy —
                                 advise patient to see her dentist.

4. General advice: Talk to the mother and answer questions
                             Refer to mothercraft/relaxation classes
                             Arrange tours of delivery suites, lectures,
                                 etc.

5. Drugs: In general, avoid prescribing in pregnancy
                                 especially in the first trimester
                                 (organogenesis)
                             Some drugs are thought to be safe:
                                 antiemetics — some are safe
                                 antibiotics — penicillins and
                                     cephalosporins
                                 anticoagulants — heparin acceptable,
                                     oral anticoagulants less safe
                                 sedatives and tranquillisers —
                                     generally 'safe' (but thalidomide
                                     was a tranquilliser thought to be
                                     safe for use in pregnancy) but if
                                     used at term can cause neonatal
                                     respiratory depression
                                 antihypertensives — methyldopa,
                                     labetalol.

HIGH-RISK SITUATIONS

Certain groups of pregnant women are recognised as being
'high-risk'.

Elderly primigravidae

Age greater than 35 at first pregnancy (note that it is age rather than
the nulliparity that matters) at risk because/from:

- increased incidence of fetal abnormality
- the baby is likely to be 'precious' — previous infertility is
  common and available time for future pregnancies is limited.

Special measures:	Amniocentesis if appropriate — 'triple' blood test avoids need for 'automatic' amniocentesis. Maternal serum AFP may also help avoid amniocentesis for Down's Book for hospital delivery Consider induction of labour at term Close fetal monitoring in labour.

Grand multiparity

Fifth or subsequent delivery (not pregnancy) at risk because/from:	Increased perinatal mortality Increased maternal mortality Maternal anaemia and general ill health Unstable fetal lie, malpresentations 'precipitate' labour Late engagement of the fetal head Postpartum haemorrhage Uterine rupture.
Special measures:	Hospital delivery with blood available Close antenatal supervision Contraceptive advice post delivery Intravenous ergometrine at delivery.

Obesity

At risk because/from:	Increased hypertension and pre- eclampsia Obstetric assessment is difficult Fat mothers produce fat (i.e. big) babies Increased operative and anaesthetic risk Increased risk of gestational DM.
Special measures:	Aim for no overall weight gain in pregnancy Hospital delivery Glucose tolerance test Use large cuff for blood pressure measurements to avoid spurious over-reading.

GENETIC COUNSELLING

Definition
Advice given to patient or family about an hereditary disorder so that they can make a rational decision about further pregnancies.

Counselling concerned with:

Psychological aspects:
  relief of guilt
  anger
  blame
  unhappiness
Correction of misconceptions
Introduction to lay organisations.

About 1 child in 40 is born with a significant malformation.

Incidence of some genetic disorders:

Heart malformation 8/1000
Severe mental retardation 3/1000
Spina bifida 3/1000
Cleft lip/palate 1/1000
Pyloric stenosis 3/1000
Neurofibromatosis 0.4/1000.

Single gene defects
3000 conditions
Risk of producing affected offspring mathematically calculated.

Dominant—fully expressed in heterozygous state, i.e. need only a single 'dose' of mutant gene to express condition.

Recessive — individual with a recessive disorder is homozygous for mutant gene and is born to normal heterozygous carrier parents.

X-linked — mutant gene carried on X chromosome. Most are X-linked recessive and not expressed in females. Male to male transmission does not occur. Males are hemizygous: if gene present it is expressed even though recessive.

Autosomal dominant:
(7/1000)

Risk of recurrence 50%
No sex predilection
Family history -ve and case a fresh
  mutation, risk to siblings nearly zero but
  affected individual transmits to half his
  offspring, e.g. Huntington's disease.

Autosomal recessive:
(2.5/1000)

Risk to siblings of affected individual =
  25%
Risk 25% in each pregnancy
Consanguinity increases risk — advise of
  hazard of marrying close relative.

X-linked recessive:
(1/1000)

Heterozygous female has 25% chance of
  having affected child (50% chance of
  having male child and 50% of males
  affected)

	Heterozygous females have normal girls
	Ultrasound scan or amniocentesis used for sexing
	X-linked gene probes make detection of affected male possible.
X-linked dominant:	Half of all children of affected females affected regardless of sex
	All of the daughters and none of the sons of an affected male will be affected.

Heterozygote detection
Important in X-linked recessive conditions: female siblings of affected boys and maternal aunts have a high risk of being heterozygotes and may have affected children, e.g. muscular dystrophy, haemophilia, Hunter syndrome (mucopolysaccharidosis), Lesch–Nyhan syndrome (hereditary hyperuricaemia).

Chromosome abnormalities
Down's sydnrome (trisomy 21)
Edward's syndrome (trisomy 18)
Patau's syndrome (trisomy 13)
Deletion syndromes (cri du chat).

Sex chromosome anomalies:	Gonadal dysgenesis or Turner's syndrome — absence of X chromosome in females
	Klinefelter's syndrome — 47, XXY
	X/linked mental retard
	Intersex states.

Fortunately, chromosome abnormalities occur only once in a family. Parental karyotypes are essential for counselling. The availability of antenatal diagnosis and selective abortion must be offered to those at risk.

ANTENATAL/IN UTERO DIAGNOSIS

Expanding field.
Relative importance greater as perinatal mortality from all causes falls.
Serious chromosome abnormalities are as common as intrapartum death with more serious long-term consequences.
In developed countries:
    30% of stillbirths
    20% of neonatal deaths
    30% of paediatric admissions
are the result of congenital disorders.

Antenatal/in utero diagnosis relies on:
- Ultrasound scans
- x-rays still occasionally have a place
- Assays of pregnancy hormones and fetal products
- Analysis of fetal tissue/blood/fluid.

Ultrasound

Indications for ultrasound scan:

Previous abnormal child
Parent with abnormality
Raised maternal serum AFP
Oligohydramnios
Polyhydramnios
Multiple pregnancy
Small or large for dates.

Conditions diagnosed by ultrasonography:

Anencephaly
Hydrocephaly
Spina bifida
Encephalocoele
Oesophageal atresia
Diaphragmatic hernia
Duodenal atresia
Jejunal atresia
Cystic fibrosis
Omphalocoele
Gastroschisis
Hydronephrosis
Urethral obstruction
Renal agenesis
Achondroplasia
Cardiac anomalies
Facial deformities
Cleft palate.

Ultrasonography may also be used to assess blood flow in the umbilicial cord and fetal aorta by means of Doppler techniques if there is concern about placental function.

X-rays
X-rays may be used to determine the position/posture of the fetal head in the breech presentation, and may be used to confirm an intra-uterine death (Spalding's sign; gas in the major blood vessels; collapse of the spine) if ultrasonography is not available.

Pregnancy hormones and fetal products
Pregnancy hormones — HCG and HPL have been used to assess fetal well- being/placental function and, along with urates, may be used to assess the progress of toxaemia of pregnancy, as may platelet level and a coagulation profile.

The 'triple test' which assays the levels of AFP, HCG and oestradiol in the maternal serum at about 16 weeks' gestation, may be used to assess the risk of the mother carrying a Down's fetus, thereby avoiding an 'automatic' amniocentesis for a mother at risk.

Alpha-fetoprotein estimations (AFP):	Main fetal serum protein during first 20 weeks
	Leaks across exposed membranes:
	    spina bifida
	    anencephaly
	    exomphalos
	Measured in maternal serum and amniotic fluid
	Sensitivity 90% for anencephaly, and 80% for NTDs
	Most useful as a screen if no ultrasound
	Liquor acetyl cholinesterase may help confirm diagnosis.

Using fetal fluids and tissues:

- Amniocentesis — liquor
- Chordocentesis — fetal blood
- Fetoscopy:
  - fetal blood
  - fetal skin
  - fetal liver biopsy
- Chorionic villus biopsy.

Amniocentesis:	Performed under ultrasound control May be performed as early as 12 weeks Usually about 15 weeks Risk of miscarriage = 0.5–2% Cell culture for chromosomes about 3 weeks May be used in third trimester to assess: fetal lung maturity (surfactant) — now mainly of historic interest — and also bilirubin levels in Rh – Ve mothers with an immunised fetus — replaced in modern practice by fetal blood sampling for bilirubin and anaemia. Fetal anaemia may also be detected by ultrasound and Doppler.
Fetoscopy:	Reducing need for this technique; more sampling being done under ultrasound control.

Performed after 18 weeks' gestation with a miscarriage rate of about 3%, plus an incidence of pre-term labour and leak of liquor.

Chorionic villus sampling (CVS):

Performed at 09–11 weeks
Trans-cervical and trans-abdominal
Allows earlier TOP
Chorion used for:
    chromosome tests
    enzyme assay
    gene probes
Current anxieties about congenital abnormalities associated with the procedure
Causes abortion in 2–3%.

Fetal tissues/blood can be sent for:

- chromosome analysis
- enzyme analysis
- haematological tests
- recombinant DNA technology.

Chromosome analysis:

Most important = aneuploidies (abnormality of chromosome number) e.g. trisomies, monosomy (Turner's).

Enzyme defects:

Inborn errors of fetal metabolism diagnosed by incubating fetal cells with specific substrates
Some may be diagnosed by metabolite collecting in liquor
Used for parents who have had an affected child, or carriers.

Fetal blood tests:

Haemoglobinopathies
Haemophilia
Christmas disease
(Being replaced by gene probe techniques).

Recombinant DNA technology:

Chromosomes separated
Gene mapping performed
Binding pattern demonstrated by special stains
Regions divided into bands
Site of gene then localised.

Antenatal care. 2: Abnormal conditions of pregnancy

Comprehensive antenatal care has developed in order to identify those women most at risk of having an abnormal outcome to their pregnancy, i.e. those women who if left alone and unattended would suffer an increased maternal and fetal mortality and morbidity.

FETAL ABNORMALITY

Fetal abnormality may present in one or more of the following ways:

- polyhydraminos
- IUGR + IUD
- breech presentation
- unstable lie
- malpresentation/abnormal lie
- disproportion
- post-maturity.

Investigations

Routine:

Ultrasound
Maternal serum alpha-fetoprotein (2nd trimester).

Special (for use when fetal abnormality is suspected):

Liquor AFP or AChE ⎫
Chromosome analysis ⎪
Fetoscopy ⎬ 2nd trimester
Fetal blood sampling (for ⎪
  haemoglobinopathies) ⎭
CVS
X-ray (may still have a place in 3rd trimester).

Management

The results of all the investigations are discussed in full with the parents, who will want to be informed about many points, including the degree of handicap, the length of survival and the chance of the abnormality recurring. Discussions with a consultant paediatrician and/or a consultant geneticist are very helpful in the presence of an abnormal result. They are given the option of continuing with or terminating the pregnancy.

Methods of termination of pregnancy
Prostaglandin TOP using a solution or gel extra-amniotically, or a solution + urea intra-amniotically (2nd trimester).
Hysterotomy (now very unusual in UK).
Some surgeons will terminate vaginally (by suction TOP) up to 18 weeks; 12–14 weeks is a more normal limit.

Genetic counselling should be offered to all couples who have had an abnormal baby. They can then be advised whether the abnormality is a 'one off' occurrence or whether there is an increased risk of recurrence. 1 in 200 live births have chromosomal abnormalities.

Amniocentesis should be offered to all women over the age of 36 years, but the mother must be advised that the procedure carries a risk of causing an abortion (variously assessed as 0.5–2.0%) and of causing fetal injury.

Triple testing for Down's syndrome
The test uses a combination of

- maternal age
- serum AFP
- unconjugated oestriol
- human HCG

to select those mothers at high risk of having a Down's baby, thus avoiding 'blanket' amniocentesis to mothers over 35 years old.

Although attractive on paper, there have been problems with application, and sensitivity, in practice, may be similar to that of amniocentesis.

Down's syndrome
Incidence: 1 in 160 live births.
Mothers >40 years have a 1 in 50 chance of having a Down's baby, rising to 1 in 20 at 45 years.
1 in 100 chance of a second Down's baby.

Spina bifida
1 in 300 risk of spina bifida, but 1 in 25 if a previous child was affected.
Amniocentesis gives a 90% overall pick-up for neural tube defects (NTD).
Ultrasound scanning is very accurate at detecting NTDs and has replaced serum AFP testing in some centres.

ANTEPARTUM HAEMORRHAGE

Antepartum haemorrhage is bleeding occurring from the genital tract after 28 weeks' gestation. It is potentially serious and may lead to the death of the mother, the baby or both. APH occurs in 5–10% of pregnancies.

Types:	Unavoidable (inevitable)
	Accidental
	Incidental.

Unavoidable

Bleeding from an abnormally situated placenta, i.e. placenta praevia.

Features:	1 in 200 births
	More common in multipara.

Four degrees of placenta praevia used to be described depending on whether or not the placenta reached or covered the os.

From a practical viewpoint the placenta in placenta praevia is now described as:

- being in the lower segment but not covering the internal os
- partially covering the os
- completely covering the os.

Accidental

Bleeding from a normally situated placenta; also called **abruptio placentae**. It may become apparent externally (i.e. revealed — 80%), or there may be no vaginal loss (i.e. concealed — 20%).

Incidental

Bleeding from any other genital tract lesion, e.g. cervical polyp, erosion.

Aetiology

Unavoidable/placenta praevia:	Idiopathic
	LSCS scar
	? poor blood supply to part of uterine body
	Large placenta (twins)
	Abnormal placenta (diffuse or succenturate lobe).
Separation may be due to:	Mechanical forces (labour)
	Formation of lower segment
	Placentitis
	Rupture of engorged venous lakes.

Accidental/abruptio placentae:	Unknown but ...... ? External version ? Fetal movements ? Increased incidence with: PET DM renal disease chronic hypertension folic acid deficiency.

Pathophysiology

Bleeding → hypovolaemic shock
Couvelaire uterus
Disseminated intravascular coagulopathy
Acute cor pulmonate (due to amniotic cellular emboli or defibrination in the pulmonary micro-circulation)
Acute renal necrosis
Acute pituitary necrosis (Sheehan's syndrome).

Signs and symptoms

Unavoidable:	Spotting in 1st and 2nd trimester PAINLESS profuse bleeding Unengaged presenting part 10% have initial cramping Uterus soft Abnormal lie Ultrasound = placenta in lower segment.

Accidental:	Uterus PAINFUL and tender Uterus irritable + or − fetal distress/IUD + or − bleeding Maternal shock.

Management

Treatment should be commenced immediately and efficiently.

Outside Hospital
Keep patient at rest, quiet and flat on left side.

Record observations fully:	Pulse BP General condition Fetal heart Vaginal loss.

Call Obstetric Flying Squad if available or dial 999.
On *NO* account do a rectal of vaginal examination.

Hospital treatment
IVI: blood (uncrossmatched blood of the patient's group + Rh factor
  if available; O Rh – ve blood if desperate) or plasma
Haemoglobin estimation
Cross match blood
FDP estimation
Serum fibrinogen level
VERY GENTLE speculum examination to exclude lower genital tract
  bleeding (facilities for an immediate LSCS must be available)
Ultrasound scan if available on labour ward, or if the time is available
  with conservative management.
Accurate diagnosis of the cause of bleeding can be very difficult.

Further management is determined by clinical situation

APH of unknown cause at or near term
Perform examination under anaesthetic ('EUA') or examination
without anaesthetic ('EWA') depending on the clinical suspicion, in
theatre with facilities for immediate LSCS available. If placenta is felt
(it feels 'boggy'), proceed to LSCS; if no placenta felt, perform ARM
to induce labour.

Unavoidable (placenta praevia)

Conservative
Before 32 weeks's gestation it is important to gain time for fetal
  maturity, therefore await the cessation of bleeding if the loss is
  light and there is no fetal distress.
Low lying placentae bleed because the lower segment is 'taken up'.
  If contractions are present tocolytics may be given.
Steroids may be given if <36 weeks' gestation to reduce the chance
  of the fetus developing respiratory distress syndrome (RDS).

Surgical
Lower segment caesarean section. (Because it may be necessary to
cut through the placenta, there is a risk of severe fetal haemorrhage
as well as the ever-present risk of major haemorrhage to the mother.)

Accidental

Conservative
Constant maternal and fetal monitoring. Both patients are at great
risk, and the first evidence of renewed bleeding may be maternal
shock and/or loss of the fetal heart. Investigations and treatment as
above.

Surgical
Induction of labour by artificial rupture of the membranes, (ARM) +
  Syntocinon

Patients with an accidental APH will often labour well, when 34 weeks' gestation or more.

LSCS recommended at 32 weeks or less.

Between 32–34 weeks, use clinical judgement to decide best mode of delivery.

Caesarean section may be required in both these conditions, even if the fetus is dead, to save the mother.

RHESUS DISEASE (HAEMOLYTIC DISEASE OF THE NEWBORN)

Rhesus incompatibility may develop when a rhesus negative woman is impregnated by a rhesus positive man and rhesus positive fetus is conceived.

Aetiology
Rhesus +ve fetal RBCs enter the maternal circulation.
Antibodiy against rhesus factor (D) is formed.
Anti-D antibodies cross the placenta.
Anti-D antibodies cause lysis of fetal RBCs.

Features
Fetal anaemia
Oedematous (hydropic) fetus
Fetal death in utero
Postnatal accumulation of fetal bilirubin
Kernicterus
First pregnancy rarely affected
Bile stained liquor.

Prevention
Injection of anti-D gamma-globulin within 72 hours of delivery, abortion or TOP in Rh –ve mothers
Screening of the mother at antenatal booking for blood group, rhesus factor and antibodies
Kleihauer–Shephard test on maternal and vaginal blood
Antibody titres at 28 and 34 weeks
The development of rhesus haemolytic disease may be detected by:
    rising anti D titres
    liquor bilirubin levels
    ultrasound scans may show evidence of fetal hydrops in
        severely affected fetuses.

Treatment
Early delivery (after 32 weeks if possible)
In utero fetal transfusion to correct the anaemia
Atraumatic delivery and third stage (to reduce the feto-maternal transfusion)
After delivery (to the infant):
    exchange transfusion
    phototherapy.

PRE-ECLAMPTIC TOXAEMIA (PET) AND ECLAMPSIA

PET is a disorder, the pathological basis of which is poorly understood, which is recognised clinically by:

- raised blood pressure
- oedema (or excess weight gain)
- albuminuria.

NB These are physical signs.
There are no symptoms of mild or moderate PET.
Of these signs, raised blood pressure is essential to the diagnosis, whilst oedema and proteinuria may or may not be present.
PET is a disease of the second half of pregnancy, and with the rare exception of molar pregnancy, should not be diagnosed before 20 weeks, when it is more likely that renal disease will be responsible for the symptoms/signs.

Classification
Mild (mildly raised BP alone)
Moderate (raised BP + oedema + /or albuminuria)
Severe (eclampsia may be imminent – v.i.). At this stage the disease becomes symptomatic.

Incidence
About 5% of all pregnancies
Increased in primigravidae
May be superimposed upon hypertension
Associated with:
      twins (2–3 times more common)
      diabetes mellitus
      hydrops fetalis
      hydatidiform mole (this is the only situation in which PET can develop before 20 weeks).

Diagnosis
Any BP >140/90 mmHg. This is an 'absolute' diagnosis.
A rise in the diastolic pressure of >20 mmHg from the pre-pregnancy/booking levels. This is a 'relative' diagnosis.

Severe PET

Features:
        Headaches
        Spots before the eyes/flashing lights
        Diplopia
        Dizziness
        Epigastric discomfort
        Vomiting
        Itchy nose.

These symptoms indicate imminent eclampsia and must be urgently treated.

However some patients are brought in as emergencies having had an eclamptic fit at home completely 'out of the blue'.

Remember that most eclamptic fits occur in the puerperium.

Aetiology
This is unknown. It is called the disease of theories as so many have been advanced to explain it. Relevant factors are thought to include:

Inadequate invasion of decidua by trophoplast
A deficiency of prostacyclin
Reduced refractoriness to the pressor effects of angiotensin II
Micro-emboli of trophoblast into the pulmonary circulation
Placental blood vessel changes + placental degeneration
? A failure of immune tolerance between the feto-placental unit and the mother
Altered renal function due to a renal vascular lesion
Reduced GFR
DIC and fibrin deposition
Reduced volume in the intra-vascular compartment.

Effect on the fetus and placenta
In utero growth retardation
In utero death
Fetal distress during labour
Fetal asphyxia
Placental changes: infarction
                  fibrosis replacing blood vessels
Raised perinatal mortality rate
Prematurity due to the natural onset of pre-term labour or iatrogenic pre-term delivery.

Management

Mild and moderate PET
Good antenatal care
Investigate 1st trimester hypertension
Rest
Sedation (of doubtful use)
Watch weight and salt intake
Induction of labour may be indicated in the interests of the fetus
There is no point in allowing labour to go beyond 38–40 weeks.

Severe fulminating PET
The threat of eclampsia is prominent here, therefore:
heavy sedation (diazepam i.v.)
hydralazine or labetalol i.v.
induction of labour or LSCS.

Complications of severe PET/eclampsia
Accidental APH
Fetal and/or maternal death.

Prophylaxis
Junior aspirin daily (75 mg) may reduce the incidence of the condition.
(CLASP trial — look up.)

Urinary suppression
Patients with moderate PET have altered renal function, and in those with severe PET oliguria may be a marked feature; tubular or cortical necrosis may occur, but very unusual.

Management
Encourage diuresis post-delivery (mannitol or frusemide)
Fluid restriction
Accurate fluid balance
Continue anti-hypertensive therapy
Continue anti-convulsant therapy.

Eclampsia
The word 'eclampsia' means to strike forth or suddenly appear, but in fact eclampsia is the end result of a gradually progressive disease: pre-eclamptic toxaemia. In eclampsia, the mother has generalised convulsions, but may also be deeply comatose. Untreated, death of the mother and fetus may result.

Incidence
Now rare in the UK.
Approximately 1/200 cases of PET
Maternal mortality worldwide: 0–17%
Fetal mortality worldwide: 10–37%
    Prevention of eclampsia by adequate management of PET, including elective early delivery, is of paramount importance. The importance of careful supervision of pre-eclamptic patients in the puerperium cannot be overstressed.
    Should eclampsia develop, it is a medical emergency which must be given the highest priority by the obstetric and midwifery team on site.

Management
The aim is to prevent maternal complications and to deliver a healthy baby:
    Involve the anaesthetist
    Establish IVI

Give diazepam 10 mg i.v.stat. to control fits (but not relied on to prevent fits)
Repeat if necessary
Give hydralazine i.v. by infusion to control blood pressure
Ensure control of airway: padded spatula in mouth; replace with plastic airway after convulsion
Mother in Trendelenberg position
Aspirate secretions/vomitus
Estimate FBC, PCV, U + Es, coagulation screen
Maintain accurate fluid balance chart
Assess the cervix: is it ripe for induction/does it suggest that the mother will deliver quickly?
If cervix unfavourable, deliver fetus by LSCS.
*Delivery/termination of the pregnancy is THE treatment for PET/eclampsia.
After delivery: continue sedation
                practise fluid restriction
                encourage diuresis prn with frusemide
                if coma persists, mannitol (an osmotic diuretic) may be required
                continue accurate fluid balance
                continue or institute anti-hypertensive treatment
                check renal function.
The authors appreciate that the management listed above may not be the same as practised at many teaching hospitals. Some prefer to use infusions of heminevrin for sedation, but caution is required here not to over-infuse the patient.

As emphasised in the introduction, get to know the management as *your* hospital and be able to explain and discuss it. 'Definitive' management is described in the *Report on Confidential Enquiries into Maternal Deaths in the United Kingdom* (latest 1985–87).

NAUSEA AND VOMITING

This is common in pregnancy and is a sign of pregnancy. It may be due to:

- HCG
- oestrogen
- oesophageal reflux (hiatus hernia).

Treatment
Reassurance that it is normal and will pass (modern practice — no medication for first trimester)
Promethazine
Antacids
Small frequent meals.

HYPEREMESIS GRAVIDARUM

Intractable vomiting severe enough to cause maternal dehydration and acidosis in pregnancy.

Features:	Pregnant
	Vomiting
	Starvation (because of nausea)
	Dehydration
	Keto-acidosis due to starvation
	Liver damage (occasionally)
	Weight loss.
Management: Exclude:	Liver disease (LFTs, etc.)
	Renal disease.
Treatment:	Intravenous fluids
	Correct electrolyte disturbance
	Parenteral vitamins
	Small bland meals
	Terminate pregnancy (very rare).

POLYHYDRAMNIOS

In the first half of pregnancy amniotic fluid is a transudate from the maternal plasma across the membranes. In the second half of pregnancy, fetal urine is added. A volume of greater than 2000 ml equals hydramnios.

Volume
10 weeks — 30 ml
20 weeks — 350 ml
30 weeks — 1000 ml
After 38 weeks the volume declines.

Composition
SG 1.008
pH 7.2
Desquamated fetal cells
Proteins (1/10 fetal serum values)
Electrolytes similar to maternal plasma.

Function
Protection from injury
Maintains temperature
Allows free movement
Prevents fetal adherence to the membranes.

The fetus drinks about 400–500 ml per day and excretes about the same amount.

If the drinking is interfered with (either prevented or reduced), e.g. by oesophageal atresia, or there is an increased urine output, hydraminos will develop.

Causes of Hydramnios
NTD
Oesophageal atresia
Duodenal atresia
Imperforate anus
Other fetal abnormality
Maternal diabetes mellitus
Multiple pregnancy.

Complications (mainly due to overdistension of the uterus)
Pain
Pre-term rupture of the membranes
Pre-term labour
Abnormal lie/malpresentation.

Treatment
Rest
Moral support
Analgesia
Antacids prn
Terminate pregnancy if fetal abnormality.

OLIGOHYDRAMNIOS

Oligohydramnios means that there is too little liquor for the stage of pregnancy.

Cause
Fetal urinary tract abnormality:
   renal agenesis
   posterior urethral valves
Placental insufficiency.

PRETERM RUPTURE OF THE MEMBRANES

This is spontaneous rupture of the membranes before 37 weeks' gestation.

Aetiology
Idiopathic
Cervical infection + infection of the adjacent membranes
   (antenatal vaginal examinations are thought to increase the risk of this)
Hydramnios.

Management
This depends on the gestation, the fetal presentation and the presence or absence of maternal pyrexia (indicating amnionitis).

After 32 weeks
   (a) Cephalic presentation:
      Perform CTG:
      — if there is fetal distress, deliver by LSCS
      — no fetal distress, await spontaneous vaginal delivery
      If there is maternal pyrexia, induce contractions
        with Syntocinon or, if the cervix is unfavourable,
        deliver by LSCS.
   (b) Any other presentation:
      Deliver by LSCS (but allow frank breech to labour)
      (Some authorities only allow breech to labour after
        34 weeks.)

Before 32 weeks
   (a) Apyrexial:
      No vaginal examination
      Steroids (to stimulate fetal surfactant production)
      Low vaginal swab
      Bed rest
      Aim to get to 32 weeks
      Tocolytics as required (debatable — one view is that
        contractions are a sign of infection, and therefore should
        not be prevented).
   (b) Pyrexial:
      Cephalic: stimulate contractions if cervix ripe or LSCS if not
      Breech: LSCS
      Fetal distress: LSCS

PRETERM LABOUR

The onset of labour before 37 weeks' gestation. Technically, before 28 weeks, effacement and dilatation of the cervix indicate a threatened abortion, but with modern neonatal intensive care 24 weeks is a better cut-off point.

Statistics
7% of all pregnancies
Fetus <1500 g most at risk (up to 85% neonatal mortality)

Causes of preterm labour
Idiopathic
Urinary tract infection
Multiple pregnancy

Hydramnios
Maternal infection/pyrexia
Surgery
Injury
Iatrogenic, as in preterm delivery for:
  PET
  renal disease
  rhesus disease
  placenta praevia
Cervical incompetence.

Prevention
Antenatal care
Shirodkar suture (for cervical incompetence) — now debatable and
  less used
Screen for urinary tract infection and treat energetically if detected.

Treatment
Tocolytic drugs, e.g.:
  ritodrine
  isoxsuprine } beta-sympathomimetic drugs
  salbutamol
  alcohol
Treat UTI if present.
  If one cannot prevent preterm labour the main problem is how to
deliver the preterm fetus.
  Vaginal delivery imposes considerable stress on the fragile preterm
fetus. The cranial contents are especially prone to damage, and for
this reason the relatively atraumatic (for the fetus) delivery by
caesarean section may be better. Cut-off points are controversial but
current opinion may be summarised as follows:

- cephalic presentation; deliver by LSCS up to 1500 g/30 weeks
- breech presentation: deliver by LSCS up to 2000 g/33 weeks*

VERY LOW BIRTH WEIGHT BABIES (UNDER 1500 G)

Approximately 6000 VLBW babies born per annum in the UK

Outcome
75% survive to discharge (this rises to 90 + % in the 1251–1500g
group).
In infants followed for one year (denominator = live births):
  — cerebral palsy rate approximately 7.5%
  — disability rate approximately 25%

* Based on published figures from Hammersmith Hospital, London

FETAL VIABILITY AND INFANT MORTALITY RATES

Fetal viability: changes over time (rates per 1000 live births):

	NNDs	Post-NNDs	Infant deaths
1975	10.6	4.8	15.4
1980	7.6	4.3	11.9
1985	5.3	3.9	9.2
1990	4.5	3.2	7.7

Infant mortality rates by birth weight: (England and Wales per 1000 live births)

All weights	7.7
Under 1000g	Over 500 (i.e. one half of all live births)
Under 1500g	257.4
Under 2500g	53.8
2500–2999g	6.3
3000–3499g	3.7
>3500g	2.7

Infant Mortality rates by social class (England and Wales per 1000 live births)

All classes	6.7
SC 1	5.6
SC 2	5.3
SC 3	6.5
SC 4	8.3
SC 5	11.2

INTRA-UTERINE GROWTH RETARDATION

This may be defined as being present when the fetal weight is less than the fifth centile for the gestational age. Although the fetus cannot be weighed in utero, the weight may be estimated from charts after measuring the bi-parietal diameter and the abdominal circumference ultrasonically.

Approximately 30–40% of low birth weight babies demonstrate IUGR. If on measuring the BPD and AC both values are reduced, symmetrical IUGR (which is early in onset) is diagnosed.

If the BPD is within the normal range for the gestational age but the AC is low, then asymmetrical IUGR is diagnosed, which is usually of late onset.

Aetiology

Maternal:	Poor nutrition
	Smoking
	Genetic/racial features.

Feto-placental: Fetal abnormality
                           Multiple pregnancy
                           Utero-placental insufficiency due to:
                               PET
                               placental infarcts
                               placental thrombosis
                               renal hypertension.

Management: Hospitalisation and rest
                           Try to identify cause
                           Correct if possible
                           Consider preterm delivery if the cause is
                               untreatable and progressive.

MULTIPLE PREGNANCY

Definition: more than one fetus is present.

Incidence (spontaneous   Twins 1 in 80 pregnancies
pregnancies):   Triplets 1 in 80^2 = 1 in 6400
                            Quads 1 in 80^3 = 1 in 51 200
                            IVF and fertility management have altered
                                these figures.

Aetiology   Rate 4 per 1000
Monozygotic   Same in all races
pregnancies: Not influenced by any known maternal
                                factors.

Dizygotic   UK rate 12 per 1000
pregnancies: Probably inherited
                            More common in older multipara
                            Peak incidence 35–40 years
                            Increased incidence with induction of
                                ovulation.

Pathological complications

Maternal: Anaemia
                            Marked uterine distension
                            Increased incidence of placenta praevia.

Fetal: Twins may be small for dates
                            Increased incidence of congenital
                                abnormality
                            Fetus papyraceus
                            Increased incidence of velamentous cord
                                insertion
                            IUGR in one twin if monozygotic.

Multiple pregnancy is at high risk for:
                              Anaemia
                              PET/eclampsia
                              Haemorrhage (ante and post-partum)
                              Uterine inertia
                              Cord prolapse
                              Premature separation of the placenta
                              Preterm labour
                              Twin to twin transfusion.

Symptoms and signs
Exagerated symptoms of normal pregnancy.
Clinical diagnosis possible in about 75% of cases:
    palpation ≥3 poles
                multiple small parts
    auscultation 2 fetal hearts
    excess weight gain that is not oedema or obesity
    polyhydramnios
    palpation of 2nd fetus in uterus after delivery of the first infant.

Additional investigations
Ultrasound scanning
(Plain abdominal X-ray)
(Expect high HPL titres).

Differential diagnosis
Single pregnancy, inaccurate dates
Polyhydramnios
Abdominal tumours (fibroids, ovarian cyst).

Management
Early diagnosis of multiple pregnancy
More frequent antenatal visits
More rest after 24 weeks
USS checks on both twins' growth rate at 28 weeks
May need tocolytics to delay labour (increased incidence of pre-term
    labour)
Hospital delivery
If possible convert second twin to cephalic presentation by external
    version after delivery of the first
Deliver the second twin as quickly as possible (within 20 minutes is a
    medico-legal guideline)
Paediatricians present at delivery
Anaesthetists present at delivery
Caesarean section for obstetric reasons only.

BREECH

A breech presentation means that the fetal buttocks ± the feet comprise the presenting part.

Types: Incomplete or frank breech: extended legs
Complete breech: knees flexed; feet above buttocks
Footling breech: one or both feet below buttocks
Knee presentation: one or both knees below buttocks.

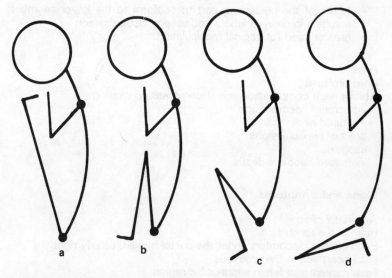

Fig. 42 The different positions of the fetus in breech presentation: (a) Frank breech (extended breech); (b) flexed breech; (c) footling breech. (d) knee presentation

The sacrum is used as the denominator, e.g. right sacrum anterior, left sacrum lateral, etc.

Incidence
3%
Varies inversely with birth weight: higher when the birth weight is lower
More common if fetus pre-term.

Aetiology

Maternal   Placental site
                           Septate/bicornuate uterus
                           Increased uterine tone
                           Oligohydramnios.

Fetal   Large head (hydrocephaly; goitre)
                           Splinting legs discourage turning.

Pathology/dangers

Breech presentation is not especially dangerous to the mother but is very dangerous to the fetus because of:

- failure of the presenting part to conform to the lower segment resulting in delay in labour and uterine incoordination
- greater need for vaginal manipulation.

Fetal
Cord prolapse
Abrupt head compression and decompression causing:
  intracranial haemorrhage
  fractured neck
  brachial plexus lesions
  asphyxia
  increased neonatal death.

Signs and symptoms

Antenatal clinic
Head in the fundus
Head causes discomfort under the costal margin, usually right
Fetal heart above the umbilicus
Fetal movements felt in supra-pubic region
Ultrasound diagnosis
X-ray diagnosis.

Labour
Abnormal presenting part felt on vaginal examination. Must be
  distinguished from anencephaly (+ face: 2 cheeks and a hole . . .)
Slow labour.
NB When palpating the breech vaginally, it is important NOT to try to
  insert a finger into the anus or vagina, although it is classically
  described that the way to distinguish the anus from the lips in a
  face presentation is to palpate the alveolar ridge in the latter.
  Feet are recognised by the short stubby toes, and distinguished
from hands by the fact that one cannot 'shake hands' with them.

Management

Antenatal:	External cephalic version is practised by some consultants X-ray pelvimetry Fetal weight estimation.
In labour:	Primigravida — consider LSCS Breech + any other abnormality (X factor) = LSCS IVI Cross match blood or save serum (check your hospital's policy) Monitor fetus and the labour very closely.
Types of delivery:	Assisted breech with forceps to after-coming head Spontaneous breech Breech extraction.

Breech presentation constitutes a risk to the fetus. Some obstetricians consider breech presentation to be a malpresentation and therefore feel that there is no place for a trial of breech labour or for artificial rupture of the membranes. In labour the progress must be constantly monitored and, if the cervix is not dilating at the optimal rate and the presenting part is not descending, then caesarean section should be performed without delay, even if the cervix is fully dilated.

UNSTABLE LIE

In this condition the fetal position keeps changing. This is normal in the first and second trimesters but puts the fetus at risk in the third trimester as there is the constant risk of cord prolapse (at the onset of labour).

Fetal death and uterine rupture may also occur.

Causes
Idiopathic
Grand multiparity
Hydramnios
Fetal abnormality
Placenta praevia
Pelvic tumours: fibroids; ovarian cysts.

Management
Admit to hospital at 37 + weeks
If labour occurs with malpresentation: LSCS

If the lie stabilises, induce at term
If unstable at term: LSCS
(Stabilising induction in the Third World may avoid LSCS).

ABNORMAL LIE

Definition: the long axis of the fetus is not parallel to the long axis of
the uterus. The lie may be:

- transverse
- oblique (cephalic or breech).

Causes
Idiopathic
Hydramnios
Fetal abnormality
Grand multiparity
Placenta praevia
Pelvic tumours
Uterine abnormality.

Management
Antenatal: observe. Admit at 37 weeks gestation.
In labour or at term: deliver by caesarean section.

DISPROPORTION

Cephalopelvic disproportion exists when the diameters of the pelvis
are smaller than the presenting diameters of the fetal head. The
matter is not as clear cut as it sounds because of moulding of the
fetal head in labour, and 'relaxation' of the maternal joints at delivery.

Aetiology

Maternal:	Small woman with small pelvis
	Pelvic tumours reducing the pelvic diameters
	Contracted pelvis:
	congenital
	rickets
	fracture injury.
Fetal:	Occipito-posterior positions
	Large baby (DM; hydrops fetalis)
	Abnormal presentations (brow or face)
	Hydrocephaly.

Management
Suspect antenatally (high head)
Trial of labour (group and save serum ready for LSCS if required)
Head descends (anticipate vaginal delivery)
No cervical dilatation or descent of the head in the presence of good
  contractions = caesarean section.

Post-caesarean section
Consider X-ray pelvimetry

FETAL ALCOHOL SYNDROME

Alcohol is a drug which passes easily across the placenta. In the past
it has been thought that a moderate intake of alcohol in pregnancy
had no adverse effects on the fetus or uterus.   Infants born to
chronic alcoholics show:

- alcohol withdrawal at birth
- low birth weight/growth retardation
- microcephaly
- anomalies of the:
  — face
  — eyes
  — heart
  — joints
  — external genitalia.

The fetal alcohol syndrome, in which the affected fetus shows
some of the major features listed above, has been described in 26%
of fetuses born to women who were considered alcoholics.
Expert opinion is divided as to the effect that lighter alcohol intakes
have on the fetus. In one British investigation an intake of 10 single
drinks per week was associated with an increased risk, of delivering
a low birth weight baby. Smaller amounts of alcohol have not been
established to be safe.
NB Alcohol has a tocolytic action if the membranes are intact.

Antenatal care. 3.
Medical conditions affecting pregnancy

NON PROTEINURIC HYPERTENSION IN PREGNANCY

Incidence: 1% of all pregnancies.

Definition: Blood pressure consistently above 140/90 mmHg, which either antedates the pregnancy or is demonstrated prior to 20 weeks' gestation. The point is to exclude pregnancy-induced hypertension (i.e. pre-eclampsia), which can be difficult as pre-eclampsia may be superimposed on chronic maternal hypertension that has not been previously diagnosed.

Causes
1. Essential (idiopathic) hypertension is most common but any of the recognised causes of hypertension may be present.
2. Examination: look especially for:
   (a) cardiac abnormality (either causing or resulting from the hypertension)
   (b) coarctation of the aorta
   (c) renal artery stenosis
   (d) retinopathy (suggestive of chronic disease).
3. Investigations:
   (a) renal function tests (don't forget urinalysis!)
   (b) urinary VMA
   (c) repeated MSUs.

In general, these patients will be admitted for observation and investigation, although some authorities suggest only the urinary VMA (to exclude phaeochromocytoma) need be performed, all other investigations being deferred until after the pregnancy.

Complications and consequences:
1. Effects of the disease on pregnancy and the fetus:

(a) increased perinatal mortality ($\times 2$ if diastolic great[...]
 100 mmHg)
(b) decreased uterine blood flow
(c) intra-uterine growth retardation
(d) placental abruption.
2. Effects of pregnancy on the disease:
 (a) super-added pre-eclampsia
 (b) medical consequences of hypertension, e.g. CVA; renal
 sequelae.

Management

1. Jointly with physician if necessary
2. Rest—either at home or in hospital
3. Antihypertensives — usually methyldopa, labetalol, hydralazine
4. Close monitoring of placental function and fetal growth
5. Consider induction at 38 weeks
6. Avoid ergometrine (hypertensive effect).

PHAEOCHROMOCYTOMA

Rare but extremely serious: mortality 50–100%.

Suggested clinically by severe intermittent hypertension but is easily missed and urinary VMA estimation is essential in all pregnant patients in whom hypertension is diagnosed antenatally and postnatally.

Complications and consequences

1. Effects of disease on pregnancy and fetus:
 (a) increased placental abruption
 (b) maternal and fetal death.
2. Effects of pregnancy on disease:
 (a) frequency and severity of hypertensive episodes are increased
 (b) greatly increased maternal mortality.

Treatment

Tumour removal is the only acceptable treatment, no matter what stage pregnancy is at.

DIABETES

Incidence: The incidence of pregnant diabetics is increasing as improved general diabetic control improves fertility.

NB Pre-conceptional counselling and tight blood sugar control at conception desirable.

Detection and diagnosis

1. If routine urinalysis on the first morning urine specimen reveals (a) heavy glycosuria (2%) on one occasion or (b) any glycosuria on two occasions an oral GTT should be performed. The other causes of glycosuria should not be forgotten:
   (a) renal glycosuria (low renal threshold)
   (b) alimentary glycosuria (rapid gut absorption causes high blood levels which exceed normal renal threshold).
2. A GTT should also be performed on any woman with a history suggestive of diabetes:
   (a) previous large babies (greater than 9 lb)
   (b) previous unexplained stillbirth/neonatal death
   (c) family history of diabetes in a first order relative
   (d) marked obesity during or following a previous pregnancy
   (e) congenital abnormality.
3. However, up to 30% of gestational diabetics do not have any features suggestive of diabetes and it has been suggested that all pregnant women should have a modified/short GTT.

Complications and consequences

1. Effects of diabetes on pregnancy and fetus:
   (a) rapid fetal growth causes large baby with attendant problems
   (b) increased intra-uterine death (particularly late on), fetal abnormality and premature labour
   (c) increased polyhydramnios
   (d) increased neonatal RDS ($\times$ 5) and hypoglycaemia
   (e) increased pre-eclampsia
   (f) increased maternal infections including pyelonephritis, vulvo-vaginal candidiasis.
2. Effects of pregnancy on disease:
   (a) pregnancy may be considered diabetogenic (for a number of reasons) particularly as it may precipitate exposure of a latent diabetic. Figure 43 illustrates the different types of diabetics encountered in obstetrics.
   (b) insulin requirements increase; diabetic control becomes more difficult
   (c) renal threshold for glucose drops from about 4 months meaning urine testing cannot be reliably used to monitor diabetic control.

Mangement

1. Good management reduces maternal and fetal risks to near normal and ideally starts in a pre-conception clinic.
2. Should be undertaken in specialist units.
3. Insulin should be increased as requirements increase.
4. Monitor by blood sugar (not urine — see above).
5. Maternal glycosylated haemoglobin levels useful for assessing quality of control.

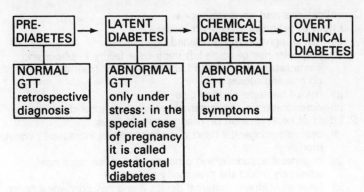

Fig. 43 Simple classification of diabetes mellitus

6. Treat any intercurrent illness, especially infection, early and vigorously.
7. Frequent monitoring of feto-placental unit.
8. Induce labour, either at 38 weeks, or, if control good and no obstetric contraindication to waiting, at term.
9. Early recourse to caesarean section if required.
10. Neonatal paediatrician should be in attendance at delivery.
11. Following delivery, the mother normally returns to her pre-pregnancy diabetic status.

HEART DISEASE

Incidence:	Less than 1% of all pregnancies. The figure is becoming even lower due to the reduction in rheumatic heart disease. Majority of patients now have congenital (rather than rheumatic) heart disease.

Diagnosis
1. Best done by a physician/cardiologist.
2. Achieved through normal means: history, examination, CXR and ECG and echocardiography.
3. Allowances should be made for the hyperdynamic circulatory state present in pregnancy (increased incidence of innocent murmurs).
4. If in doubt, the patient should be managed as if she had heart disease, and re- examined 6 weeks postnatally, a definite diagnosis reached and the patient informed.

Complications and consequences
1. Effect of pregnancy on heart disease:
   (a) risk of right and/or left sided heart failure
   (b) particular risk of acute left ventricular failure in labour and immediately after due to 'autotransfusion' from the contracting uterus
   (c) risk of bacterial endocarditis
   (d) deterioration in the maternal cardiac functional disability.
2. Effect of heart disease on pregnancy and fetus:
   (a) cyanotic congenital heart disease results in increased perinatal mortality
   (b) in general acyanotic and other heart disease does not adversely effect the pregnancy or fetus
   (c) fetus may inherit maternal defect if she has congenital heart disease.

Management
1. Jointly with a cardiologist.
2. If cardiac failure develops admit and treat vigorously.
3. Treat concurrent disease (especially anaemia) vigorously.
4. Beware pre-eclampsia (imposes even greater strain on heart).
5. Allow spontaneous labour if possible and then expedite delivery, possibly with use of elective forceps.
6. Prophylactic antibiotics as required.
7. Avoid ergometrine and oxytocics.
8. If cardiac failure does develop, treat with:
   (a) position — sit patient up if possible
   (b) frusemide
   (c) oxygen
   (d) venesection (actual or tourniquets).
9. Consider possibility of elective mitral valvotomy during the pregnancy.
   Don't forget rare but very serious cardiomyopathy of pregnancy.

ANAEMIA

Incidence: Commonest medical disorder affecting pregnancy. Incidence figures vary with definition and where study is done.

Definition
1. Pregnancy produces a state of haemodilution which may result in apparent but not true anaemia.
2. Iron (and other haematological) requirements are greatly increased in pregnancy, and therefore reduced maternal stores occur commonly but without progressing to frank anaemia.
3. It is therefore difficult to say whether a low measured haemoglobin in pregnancy reflects haemodilution, true anaemia or both.

4. It is correspondingly difficult to set a lower limit of normal for the haemoglobin in pregnancy. In practice the following figures are used:
   (a) haemoglobin less than 10–11 g/dl represents anaemia
   (b) haemoglobin between 11–13 g/dl: possible anaemia, possibly haemodilution, possibly both; requires investigation and follow-up.

Causes and diagnosis
1. The causes of anaemia in pregnancy are the same as those in non-pregnant women: in this country nutritional iron deficiency anaemia is the commonest cause of anaemia in pregnancy.
2. Diagnosis is usually by routine haemoglobin estimation, but patient may also present with the classical clinical features of anaemia (especially murmurs).
3. Investigation:
   (a) usually the blood film and/or indices will suggest iron deficiency which can be accepted as the diagnosis.
   (b) further investigation if required includes:
       (i) serum iron
       (ii) TIBC and ferritin
       (iii) serum folate/B_{12}
       (iv) stool for ova, cysts and parasites, and occult blood
       (v) remember sickle testing in African and Asian patients
       (vi) Hb electrophoresis for haemoglobinopathies.

Complications and consequences
1. Effect of disease on pregnancy and fetus:
   (a) increased perinatal mortality if Hb less than 9 g/dl
   (b) intra-uterine growth retardation
   (c) increased incidence of pre-eclampsia
   (d) less reserve for haemorrhage in or after labour
   (e) inadequate uterine contraction
   (f) PPH.
2. Effect of pregnancy on anaemia:
   (a) aggravation of anaemia (haemodilution and haemorrhage)
   (b) further depletion of iron stores.

Management
1. Prophylactic iron (and folic acid) from 12 weeks, not started before so that it cannot be implicated in any fetal abnormality.
2. Treatment of cause if identified.
3. Parenteral iron is rarely needed and infusion should be avoided if possible because of the risk of precipitating cardiac failure, allergic reaction, skin staining, etc.

URINARY TRACT DISEASE

Urinary tract infections

1. Pregnancy predisposes to urinary tract infection by causing atonic distended ureters which occur because of:
   (a) partial ureteric obstruction by the gravid uterus
   (b) the hormones present during pregnancy (especially progesterone) causing smooth muscle relaxation.
2. 6% of pregnant women have asymptomatic bacteriuria on routine investigation. Initial treatment should be with amoxycillin or equivalent.
3. Failure to treat bacteriuria or recurrence may result in acute pyelonephritis and preterm labour:
   (a) varies clinically from a mild malaise to a severe infection with high pyrexia and rigors which may result in premature labour, intra-uterine death or permanent maternal renal damage
   (b) treatment:
      (i) antibiotics
      (ii) lower temperature — paracetamol, tepid sponging
      (iii) plenty of fluids.

Other renal disease

1. Relevance to pregnancy depends on presence or absence of associated hypertension:
   (a) hypertension present: mother and fetus subject to all the complications of hypertension in pregnancy (q.v.)
   (b) hypertension not present: little effect either on mother and fetus or on the renal disease itself.
2. Investigation, diagnosis and management are the same as for non-pregnant patients.

LIVER DISEASE

Vascular spiders and palmar erythema occur in pregnancy and do not suggest liver disease, but reflect the high levels of circulating oestrogens.

Pathology of the liver in pregnancy is rare (and 50% of that which does occur is viral hepatitis). Classification is as follows.

1. Liver disease related to pregnancy:
   (a) acute fatty liver of pregnancy (very rare but usually fatal)
   (b) recurrent intrahepatic cholestasis of pregnancy (rare but usually mild disorder)
   (c) liver disease associated with hyperemesis
   (d) liver disease associated with eclampsia.
2. Liver disease not related to the pregnancy (i.e. coincidental):
   (a) includes all the usual liver diseases
   (b) viral hepatitis and gall stones commonest
   (c) treatment is essentially unaltered by the pregnancy.

THYROID DISEASE

Note: Apart from the FTI and free serum thyroxine, standard thyroid investigations are of little use in pregnancy because of the 'pseudohyperthyroid' state induced by the pregnancy.

Simple goitre
Increased iodine requirements in pregnancy may produce a goitre or cause a pre- existence goitre to enlarge.

Hyperthyroidism
1. Severe hyperthyroidism impairs fertility and is therefore rarely seen in pregnancy; if pregnancy does occur, there is an increased incidence of abortion, perinatal mortality and pre-eclampsia.
2. Graves' disease may stimulate fetal hyperthyroidism, possibly due to LATS crossing the placenta.
3. Milder degrees of hyperthyroidism properly treated result in minimal risk to mother or fetus
4. Main risk is from over-enthusiastic treatment with anti-thyroid drugs so rendering the mother hypothyroid (q.v.) and/or the fetus hypothyroid resulting in cretinism. Other treatment modalities are seldom if ever used in pregnancy.

NB Large fetal goitres can produce deflexion of the head leading to disproportion in labour.

Hypothyroidism
1. Impairs infertility and therefore rarely seen in pregnancy.
2. If present may cause abortion and premature labour.
3. Well-controlled patients on thyroxine may need increased thyroxine during the pregnancy.

PELVIC MASSES

Fibroids
1. Usually diagnosed in early pregnancy (if not before).
2. Complications:
   (a) pre-pregnancy — infertility
   (b) increased abortion rate
   (c) red degeneration of pregnancy: caused by obstruction to venous outflow: treatment is conservative
   (d) obstruction of labour: rare as fibroids are normally carried upwards as lower segment forms: cervical fibroids may require caesarean section (avoid myomectomy)
   (e) increased postpartum haemorrhage.

Ovarian masses
1. Majority are benign.
2. Complications:

    (a) may be subject to the normal complications of ovarian masses:
        (i)   rupture
       (ii) torsion
     (iii) bleeding
    (b) may cause obstruction of labour.

3. Management: large tumours (greater than 6–10 cm) should be removed, ideally at 16 weeks' gestation.

Intrapartum care. 1: Normal delivery

Labour is the process whereby the fetus, placenta and membranes are expelled from the mother. It represents the period of greatest risk to both mother and fetus, and medical management reflects this. It is also the emotional climax of pregnancy. Modern trends to humanise labour wards reflect a new awareness of this fact.

Modern obstetrics is capable of providing both safe and satisfying care for the great majority of pregnant women.

Be prepared to discuss the findings of the Parliamentary Select Committee (1992) on a return to midwifery-led care to pregnant women, away from hospitals and consultant teams.

PHYSIOLOGY OF NORMAL LABOUR

Initiation
1. Not fully understood. Overcomes progesterone effect.
2. Main trigger fetal rather than maternal.
3. May involve fetal cortisol.
4. Once initiated, labour appears to be self-perpetuating.
5. Prostaglandins now thought to be involved.

Mechanism of Labour
This is the technical name for the mechanics of the process and can be divided into various parts:
1. *Descent and engagement:*
   The fetal head descends and engages the maternal pelvis, usually in the transverse diameter (i.e. in the occipito-lateral position).
2. *Flexion and internal rotation:*
   Further contractions increase the flexion of the fetal head and cause further descent: as the fetal head descends, the muscles of the pelvic floor provide a 'channel' which causes the head to rotate through 90°, to bring the occiput anteriorly, so that it lies under the maternal symphysis pubis (internal rotation).
3. *Extension and delivery of the head:*
   Extension of the flexed fetal head, which is by now in the lowest part of the birth canal, results in its delivery.

4. *External rotation of the head and delivery of the body:*
The shoulders (which also enter the pelvis in the transverse diameter) descend and rotate through 90° to allow their delivery in the AP diameter. As they rotate they cause the already delivery head to rotate through a further 90° (external rotation/restitution). The anterior shoulder then slides out from under the pubis and the body is born by lateral flexion.

DIAGNOSIS, STAGES AND MANAGEMENT OF LABOUR

The onset of labour is defined as the beginning of regular (i.e. at least one every 10 minutes) painful contractions. Other associated events may assist in the diagnosis, but are not on their own diagnostic:
1. Show — passage of bloodstained mucus, not associated with vaginal examination
2. Spontaneous rupture of the membranes ('waters breaking')
3. Cervical dilatation of greater than 2 cm.

Stages of Labour

First stage: Onset of labour of full cervical dilatation (average duration: primigravida 8–10 h; multigravida 6–8 h); may be divided into latent and active phases.

Second stage: Full cervical dilatation to delivery of the fetus: time limits may be set, often that second stage should not last more than 2 hours. Be aware of the guidelines in your hospital. Delivery of child.

Third stage: ~~Delivery of fetus to~~ delivery of the placenta and membranes: routinely actively managed and typically lasts 5–10 minutes.

Management of labour

The majority of patients are delivered in hospital and therefore require:
1. Admission
2. Brief history and examination (assuming adequate antenatal care)
3. Routine shaving and enemas are not required but a bath or shower is recommended.

Monitoring of maternal and fetal well-being:
1. Maternal well-being:
   (a) mental state

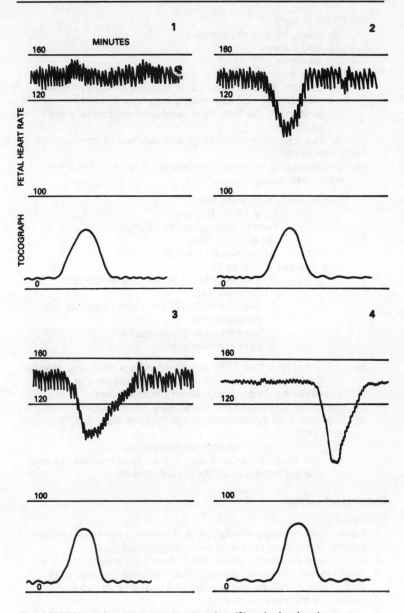

Fig. 44 (1) Normal response to a contraction; (2) early deceleration; (3) variable deceleration; (4) late deceleration and reduced beat-to-beat variability

    (b) Physical state:
       (i) pulse, BP and temperature
      (ii) fluid balance
     (iii) urinalysis
    (c) Progress of the labour:
       (i) cervical dilatation (should be approx. 1 cm/h or better) —
          mothers may be assessed 2-hourly or 4-hourly
      (ii) descent of the fetal head (assessed abdominally and
          vaginally)
     (iii) uterine activity: frequency and duration of contractions.
2. Fetal well-being:
    (a) fetal heart rate (monitor continuously if 'at risk' fetus for
       signs of distress):

       Normal cardiotocograph trace:
                 Rate 120–160/min
                 Beat-to-beat variation >5/min
                 No decelerations
                 Accelerations present
       Fetal distress indicated by:
                1. Tachycardia >160/min especially with
                   decelerations
                2. Bradycardia <120/min and especially with
                   decelerations
                3. Marked early decelerations
                4. Late decelerations

   but: note that less than 50% of fetuses with a heart rate change
      suggestive of distress will actually have distress as
      assessed by Apgar score/blood pH at delivery.
    (b) meconium staining of the liquor: may be unreliable
    (c) fetal blood pH (undertaken where facilities exist if CTG
       abnormal)
       (i) most invasive, but also most reliable index
      (ii) fetal blood pH of less than 7.2 suggests severe distress
         and indicates a need for urgent delivery.

Conduct of Labour

First stage
  1. Advantages of maternal mobility and freedom from unnecessary
     medical monitoring are being increasingly recognised.
  2. Allow bland oral fluids. Some units allow light snacks.
  3. Antacids may be given regularly, but more use is made of H_2
     antagonists to reduce gastric acidity if anaesthesia required.
  4. Encourage frequent micturition.
  5. Dehydration may require parenteral fluids; keto-acidosis does
     require parenteral fluids. No longer give dextrose; give
     Hartmann's solution.

6. Allow mother to adopt her own posture.
7. Provide analgesia as required.

Second stage
1. Allow mother to push when she wants (traditionally was only encouraged to push with contractions).
2. Monitor fetal heart rate after each contraction (if continuous trace not available).
3. Provide analgesia as required.
4. Delivery procedure:
   (a) strict asepsis
   (b) empty bladder
   (c) usually occurs with mother supine or left lateral but actual position does not matter provided the attendant:
       (i) can control the fetal head
       (ii) has access to the fetal mouth and nose (to aspirate)
       (iii) can 'protect' the maternal perineum.
5. Episiotomy should be performed if indicated.
6. Once delivered, the baby must be kept warm.
7. The cord should be cut between clamps once the pulsations have ceased.

Third stage
1. Now virtually always actively managed.
2. Syntometrine (0.5 mg ergometrine and 5 units Syntocinon) given i.m. with the anterior shoulder (NB ergometrine contraindicated in hypertensive patients and some cardiac cases). (Reduces the incidence of postpartum haemorrhage.)
3. Unclamp placenta. Await placental separation (and descent into vagina) as indicated by:
   (a) uterus becoming hard and globular
   (b) uterus appearing to rise in abdomen
   (c) further descent of the cord (clamp placed on cord at introitus can be used as marker).
4. Deliver placenta and membranes by controlled cord traction.
5. Weigh placenta and membranes and check they are intact.
6. Estimate maternal blood loss.
7. Assess maternal condition: pulse, blood pressure, uterine size, vaginal loss.
8. If required, carry out perineal repair as soon as possible.

EPISIOTOMY

Perineal incision under local (or general) anaesthesia to facilitate delivery. It has become a controversial procedure in normal deliveries, but there are some established indications for its use.

Indications (see note above):

1. Incipient tearing of the perineum (on the premise that a cut is easier to repair than a tear; and to avoid 3rd degree tears). Tears reported as less painful.
2. 'Rigid' perineum causing second stage delay.
3. Fetal prematurity (fetal head is especially vulnerable).
4. In preparation for vaginal procedures, e.g. forceps delivery.
5. Occipito-posterior position delivery.
6. Breech delivery.
7. Previous vaginal surgery.
8. Fetal distress in 2nd stage.

Complications

1. Extension, often towards the anal margin, potentially resulting in third degree tearing (avoid with 'J' shaped incision).
2. Intravaginal extension.
3. Subsequent dyspareunia.
4. Complications of any surgical procedure, in particular:
   (a) profuse haemorrhage
   (b) infection.

ANALGESIA (FOR NORMAL DELIVERY)

1. Marked reductions in the need for analgesia can be achieved by natural childbirth techniques including maternal relaxation and understanding of the process of labour.
2. Drugs:
   (a) inhalational:
       entonox (safe and generally available) 50% O_2/50%N_2O
   (b) parenteral:
       pethidine: widely used, especially in the first stage, but has problem that if used within 4 hours of delivery can cause neonatal respiratory depression requiring Narcan (naloxone) for reversal. Small doses i.v. very useful.
3. Anaesthesia:
   (a) general: not appropriate to normal delivery
   (b) regional: epidural anaesthesia may lead to increased forceps deliveries; pudendal block; caudal block
   (c) local (field) anaesthesia: perineal infiltration with lignocaine, e.g. in preparation for episiotomy.
4. 'Non-medical' analgesia:
   (a) psychoprophylaxis — very important, combined with education of the mother at antenatal classes
   (b) hypnosis.

Intrapartum care. 2. Abnormal delivery

INDUCTION OF LABOUR

Induction of labour is the artificial initiation of uterine contractions by medical and/or surgical means.

Medical: Prostaglandin E_2: (a) oral
                                                      (b) vaginal
                        Syntocinon by intravenous infusion (but only after rupture of membranes).

Surgical: Amniotomy (ARM: artificial rupture of the membranes) either forewaters or hindwaters
                      Sweeping the membranes — digital stimulation of the lower segment/cervix.

'Natural' methods — nipple stimulation and intercourse.

Indications for induction

Although the indications for induction may be maternal or fetal, often they overlap, and here they are listed together:

Pre-eclampsia
Eclampsia
Post-maturity
Abruptio placentae
Placental insufficiency/IUGR
Rhesus disease
Intra-uterine death
Hydramnios
Amnionitis
Non pre-eclamptic hypertensive disorders
Diabetes mellitus
Elderly primigravidae at term.

Contraindications

Absolute: Placenta praevia
                          Abnormal lie
                          Known contracted pelvis.

Relative: High presenting part
                          Previous LSCS
                          Breech presentation.

Induction is likely to fail in the presence of an unripe cervix.
   Bishop's score is occasionally used to 'score' the ripeness of the
cervix:
Ripe = cervix soft
         cervical os anterior
         cervix fully effaced
         cervical os 2 cm dilated
         presenting part 1 or 2 cm below the ischial spines
Unripe (unfavourable for induction) =
         cervix firm
         cervical os posterior
         cervix 40–50% effaced (about 2–3 cm long)
         cervix closed
         presenting part 1 or 2 cm above the ischial spines.
   It is possible to ripen the cervix (i.e. make it more favourable for
induction) by giving prostaglandin E_2 tablets, pessaries or gel
vaginally, or the tablets orally.

Complications: Failed induction → caesarean section
                          Fetal distress (caution when inducing for
                             IUGR; LSCS may be better)
                          Rupture of scarred uterus
                          Rupture of multigravid uterus (rupture of
                             the primigravid uterus is very rare)
                          Placental detachment
                          Rupture of vasa praevia
                          Cord prolapse
                          Amniotic fluid embolus (rare; associated
                             with oxytocics immediately after ARM or
                             with intact membranes)
                          Amnionitis.

ABNORMAL LABOUR

Abnormal labour occurs when the process of labour is not
proceeding in the normal way, i.e. the cervix is not dilating at 1 cm
per hour or more, and the presenting part is not descending.

Although there are many causes, this may be regarded as the 'final common pathway' which is common to all abnormal labours.

Causes (traditionally defined as a fault of one or more of the following):

                                    The passenger
                                    The passages
                                    The powers (forces).

The passenger: Malpresentation
                                    Malposition
                                    Hydrocephaly
                                    Fetal tumour
                                    Macrosomia (diabetic pregnancies)
                                    Hydrops fetalis
                                    Locked twins
                                    Siamese twins/monsters.

The passages: Pelvic tumour
                                    Pelvic contracture: inlet
                                                        mid-cavity
                                                        outlet
                                    Low placenta
                                    Cervical fibrosis/stenosis
                                    Vaginal septum
                                    Rigid perineum.

The powers (force) —   Incoordinate uterine activity (primigravidae)
inadequate: Maternal exhaustion — dehydration +
                                        keto-acidosis.

TRIAL OF LABOUR

A trial of labour may be indicated where cephalo-pelvic disproportion is suspected. The obstetrician is testing the ability of the fetus to pass through the pelvis. In the past, the term trial of labour was further subdivided to be more specific about which feature was actually being tested. Thus the terms 'trial of inlet', 'trial of scar', 'trial of breech' were recorded.

Nowadays, the term trial of labour implies that the progress of labour is going to be closely assessed using the parameters of cervical dilatation and descent of the presenting part in the presence of good uterine contractions. The term implies that should labour not progress normally, the fetus will be delivered by caesarean section.

Cephalo-pelvic disproportion
See p. 162

MALPOSITION

Malposition refers to abnormal positions of the occiput in a vertex presentation:

- occipito-posterior positions
- occipito-lateral positions (deep transverse arrest).

Occipito-posterior (OP)

The occiput is posterior to the pelvic transverse diameter. Although it may be suspected before the onset of labour (non-engaged head at term), or in early labour (slow progress), many OP positions are not recognised until well into the labour.

Aetiology
Fetal: Extended head — goitre
                               increased tone causing
                               neck extension.

Maternal: Anthropoid pelvis
                               Grande multipara — lax muscles.

Pathophysiology: Poor stimulation of lower segment
                               Non-engagement of head
                               Delay 1st stage
                               Uterine inertia
                               Maternal distress
                               Fetal distress
                               Deep transverse arrest if rotates from OP
                               Delay 2nd stage.

Signs and symptoms   Flattened abdomen/uterus
Antenatal: Fetal limbs easily palpable
                               Non-engaged head (especially
                                 primigravidae)
                               Fetal heart loudest in flanks.

In labour: Posterior fontanelle (identified by 3 sutures)
                                 in posterior pelvis
                               Severe backache
                               Delay 1st stage
                               Retention of urine.

Management   There is nothing active that one can do
Antenatal: except hope for normal labour with
                                 rotation to an occipito-anterior position.

In labour: Ensure good contractions (Syntocinon prn)
                               Epidural analgesia or good sedation

Close fetal monitoring
No progress 1st stage — LSCS
No progress in 2nd stage — wide
 episiotomy; forceps, either deliver OP or
 rotate with Kiellands to OA and deliver
 LSCS
Ventouse also used.

Complications
Maternal: Distress — emotional and metabolic
                             Anaesthetic hazards
                             Infection
                             Haemorrhage (vaginal vault laceration)
                             Thrombo-embolism
                             Complications of LSCS:
                                 wound haematoma
                                 UTI
                                 wound abscess
                                 (ureteric damage).

Fetal: Distress
                             Cord prolapse
                             Intrapartum death
                             Neurological damage.

Deep Transverse Arrest
The fetal head is stuck in an occipito-lateral position, in the
 transverse diameter of the outlet, between the ischial spines.
Transverse arrest may occur higher, in the mid-cavity of the pelvis.

Aetiology
Deflexion of the fetal head
Poor uterine contractions
Inadequate channelling of the fetal head by the pelvic floor (as
 happens with a relaxed pelvic floor under epidural).

Pathophysiology
As for OP positions.

Management
1st stage: Ensure good contractions with oxytocics
                             If labour becomes arrested, i.e. there is no
                                 further cervical dilatation, proceed to
                                 caesarian section.

2nd stage: Kielland's rotational forceps
                             Ventouse (vacuum) extraction
                             Caesarean section.

MALPRESENTATIONS

A malpresentation is any presentation other than by the vertex. This includes:

- breech presentation
- brow presentation
- face presentation
- shoulder presentation.

Brow

Incidence
1:2000 deliveries.

Diagnosis
High head
Large presenting diameter
Orbital ridges palpable on vaginal examination.

Management
Vaginal examination to exclude cord prolapse
Caesarean section.
  A brow presentation is unstable and may spontaneously flex in labour, or may further extend to become a face presentation, which if it is mento-anterior (see below) can be delivered vaginally.

Outcome
Safest by caesarean section, but can occasionally deliver vaginally.

Face

Incidence
1:500 deliveries.

Diagnosis
High head
Orbital ridges, mouth and gums palpable + chin on vaginal examination.

Management
Determine the position of the chin, the denominator in this presentation.
Mento-posterior and mento-lateral: caesarean section.
Mento-anterior: as for normal labour but anticipate delay and beware of cord prolapse. Perform a wide episiotomy and forceps delivery if required.
Kielland's forceps for rotation may occasionally be required.

Fetal outcome
Oedematous face
Bruised face
Sucking initially difficult.

Shoulder

Incidence
Not known.

Diagnosis
Arm in the vagina on examination.

Anticipate when:	Transverse lie
	Lax uterus
	Placenta praevia (partial)
	Multiple pregnancy
	Hydramnios.

Management
Deliver by caesarean section.

PRESENTATION AND PROLAPSE OF THE CORD

| *Presentation:* | A loop of cord lies below the presenting part; the membranes are intact. |
| *Prolapse:* | The cord is below the presenting part and the membranes have ruptured. It occurs in about 1:400 deliveries. |

Aetiology
Long cord
Poorly fitting presenting part (e.g. in malpresentations)
Malposition
Hydramnios
Twins (especially the 2nd cord).

Diagnosis
The cord may be visible at the introitus
Vaginal examination.

Complications
Fetal death.

| *Management* | |
| Dead fetus: | Continue vaginal delivery unless shoulder presentation which requires either a destruction operation on the fetus or a caesarean section. |

Live fetus:

Keep hand in the vagina
Monitor fetal heart
Keep presenting part off the cord
Raise end of the bed
Lay mother on her side or knee–elbow
    position
Caesarean section
(Catheterisation + filling of the bladder has
    also been described if mother needs
    moving a distance).

If cord prolapse occurs in the second stage, a rapid forceps delivery
is performed.

MULTIPLE PREGNANCY

See pp. 157–158.

TECHNIQUES OF ABNORMAL DELIVERY

Forceps

Forceps deliveries either involve rotating the fetal head or they do
not. The former are called rotational and the latter straight forceps
deliveries.

Types of forceps
Kielland's (rotational forceps)
Wrigley's (outlet/low cavity forceps)
Neville Barners'
Haig Ferguson's
Simpson's.

Indications
Delay in the 2nd stage (ensure good contractions first)
OP positions
Deep transverse arrest
Fetal distress
Maternal distress
Maternal hypertensive disorders
Maternal cardiac disorders
Maternal pulmonary disorders
After-coming head in breech.

Prerequisites
Cervix fully dilated
Bladder empty
Membranes ruptured
Head must be engaged with none palpable per abdomen
Denominator must be identified

Uterine contractions must be effective
Adequate anaesthesia
Episiotomy.

Anaesthesia
Perineal infiltration
Pudendal block
Caudal block
Epidural or spinal
General.

Complications
Maternal: Lacerations of genital tract (cervical tear,
                               3rd degree tear, etc.)
                             Haemorrhage
                             Shock
                             Retention of urine
                             Failed forceps (proceeding to caesarean
                               section).

Fetal: Cephalhaematoma
                             Facial palsy
                             Intra-cranial haemorrhage with neurological
                               damage, or death
                             Bruising.

Forceps delivery is attended by increased maternal and fetal mortality
and morbidity. No longer are 'high' (i.e. the fetal head is high in the
pelvic cavity above the ischial spines) forceps deliveries acceptable in
modern British obstetric practice. Caesarean section is safer and
therefore preferred.

Ventouse extraction

Indicв Indications: ⎫
Prerequisites: ⎭   As for forceps delivery.

Complications
Maternal:
As for forceps delivery.

Fetal:
   Cephalhaematoma (which resolves spontaneously)
   Ulceration of the scalp
   Tentorial tears/intracranial haemorrhage

Failed Ventouse extraction is an indication for caesarean section, *not*
a trial of forceps.
   It is very important that the cup of the Ventouse is placed as close
as possible to the occiput so as to assist flexion of the head.

Caesarean section

Caesarean section is the delivery of the fetus through the abdominal wall. It may be an elective or an emergency procedure.

Indications
Disproportion
Placenta praevia
Prolonged labour
Severe PET/eclampsia
Diabetes mellitus
Rhesus disease
Malpresentation
Cord prolapse
Fetal distress
Multiple pregnancy
Poor obstetric history.

Incidence
4–20%.

Types

Classical:	Mid-line uterine incision.
Lower segment:	Transverse or vertical incision in the lower segment.

Abdominal incisions
Pfannenstiel
Sub-umbilical mid-line.

Complications
Those common to any anaesthetic
Mendelson's syndrome
Haemorrhage
Wound infection
Endometritis
Pulmonary embolism
Respiratory tract infection
Scar rupture in subsequent pregnancies.

Primary postpartum haemorrhage

Definition:	Maternal bleeding in excess of 500 ml occurring within 24 hours of delivery.

Note: Serious and potentially lethal
    Blood loss tends to be underestimated at delivery.

Incidence:	Varies: 3–10% Has increased in recent years.

Causes:	Failure of uterus to contract due to:
	   retained products/placenta
	   uterine atony
	   trauma to:
	     uterus
	     cervix
	     vagina
	     perineum.

Predisposing factors:	Overdistended uterus (e.g. twins) Grand multiparity ('baggy uterus') Instrumental delivery Use of oxytocics — must be continued after 3rd stage.
Management Prevention:	Antenatal iron therapy Active management of the 3rd stage using Syntometrine and controlled cord traction to deliver the placenta.
Treatment of *established PPH:*	Set up IVI and cross match blood Call anaesthetist CVP line and indwelling urinary catheter Give ergometrine 0.5 mg i.v. (unless contraindicated) — may give prostaglandin $F_2\alpha$ into myometrium Transfuse — always assume that the blood volume lost is greater than you think, and replace blood as quickly as it is lost.

Treatment of specific causes:

Massage uterus
  ('rub up a contraction') } for atony or clot retention
Syntocinon drip
Ensure no lacerations
Bimanual compression of uterus
Do clotting screen and, if evidence of DIC, involve haematologist in management — fresh frozen plasma
Hysterectomy is the last resort.

Retained placenta (or part of): remove (under GA).
Tears/lacerations: repair under local/general anaesthesia.

Complications:	Death Renal failure Sheehan's syndrome (rare but famous) — pituitary necrosis Postpartum anaemia.

The puerperium

Definition: The time taken for the mother to recover from the effects of childbirth and delivery This does not imply a return to the precise pre-pregnant state. It lasts for about 6–7 weeks as judged by loss of lochia.

PHYSIOLOGY OF THE PUERPERIUM

The uterus: Bulk reduces by involution following withdrawal of oestrogens:

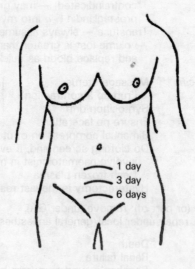

1 day
3 day
6 days

Fig. 45 Uterine involution following delivery; fundal height at 1,3 and 6 days post-delivery

—by day 1: 18 weeks' size
—by day 3: 16 weeks' size
—by day 6: 14 weeks' size
—day 10–12: not palpable abdominally
(but note that it may never
return to its nulliparous
size).

Uterine contractions, expelling cast-off
debris, give rise to after pains (which are
often exacerbated by breast feeding).
Cervix takes on its split parous
appearance.

Lochia:

Defined as the uterine discharge following
delivery.
Often heavier after breast feeding.
Normally lasts for 3–6 weeks:
— first few days — mainly blood
— the next 7–10 days — serosanguinous
— the remaining time till cessation —
yellowish.

Consists of red blood cells, white cells,
decidua and fibrinous products.

Normal vaginal bacterial flora re-
established in 72 hours: includes *Esch. coli*,
staphylococci and *Clostridium welchii*.

Ovarian function:

Returns as prolactin levels fall
New pregnancy rare in less than 6 weeks.

Urinary tract:

Micturition should occur within 12 hours of
delivery
Diuresis occurring over the next 2–5 days
removes most of the excess fluid
retained during pregnancy.

Blood:

Haemoglobin level is stable by 5th day
postpartum (but see below for when to
do postpartum haemoglobin)
Leucocytosis returns to normal.

Gastrointestinal tract:

Defaecation should occur by day 3
(depending on whether enema given or
not)
Constipation is common.

Mental state:	Elation may give way to '5th day blues" (possible due to hormonal changes).

AIMS OF PUERPERAL CARE

Restoration of optimum maternal health (including prevention, or detection if necessary, of bleeding, sepsis and thrombo-embolism)

Achievement of optimum infant health

Establishment of bonding

Establishment of lactation

Education of the mother

Rapid return of the mother to normal life.

ROUTINE PUERPERAL CARE

Observations:	Temperature; pulse and blood pressure Uterine size daily Lochia daily Urine output Bowels Haemoglobin (day 5) (but note that evidence suggests day 1 haemoglobin approximates best to 6 week haemoglobin)
Analgesia:	For after pains, episiotomy, caesarean section wound.
Sedation:	If unable to sleep.

Perineum:	Removal of sutures not needed provided absorbable sutures used for episiotomy repair.
	
	Pain relief:
	       air ring
	       analgesics
	       local heat
	       ultrasound
	       ice packs for oedema
	       local creams/foams.

General:	Postnatal exercises Attention to diet Psychological support Education in mothercraft.

Infant feeding:

Breast feeding versus bottle feeding: current medical opinion tends to favour breast feeding. If bottle feeding is intended, lactation may be actively suppressed, but current practice is to provide analgesia only for engorged breasts.

Advantages of breast feeding:

- more easily digested by the infant, simple, safe and free
- the infant's chance of gastrointestinal and possibly other infections is reduced (passive immunity)
- contains the right things in the right amounts
- overfeeding is almost impossible
- uterine involution is assisted
- the incidence of subsequent breast carcinoma is possibly reduced if mother less than 20 years old
- reduced incidence of eczema in infant.

Discharge:

May be early (48 hours or less) or longer. Advantages of early discharge:

- rapid bed throughput, so allowing increased percentage of hospital deliveries
- reduced risk of maternal/neonatal hospital acquired infection
- some obstetric units are dingy and depressing places
- early discharge is often preferred by the patient.

Advantages of longer lying-in period:

- mother goes home more rested
- more time is available to educate the mother
- lactation can be better established
- longer relief from the housework
- medical problems developing in the mother or infant after 48 hours are more likely to be noticed.

Postnatal visit

Usually done at 6 weeks, patients usually prefer to visit GP rather than hospital.

Mother: History of blood loss or pain
Examine weight and blood pressure
Examine breasts:
  nipples
  masses
Examine pelvic organs:
  episiotomy for healing
  state of cervix
  uterine size and mobility
  smear test if not done within 3–5
    years (depending on local practice)
Contraception.

Infant: Full history, especially:
  feeding
  weight gain
Examination, especially:
  umbilicus
  circumcision if present
  neurological development.

PUERPERAL COMPLICATIONS

Puerperal pyrexia

Definition: Any febrile condition occurring in a woman in whom a temperature of 38°C or more has occurred within 14 days after confinement or miscarriage.

Causes: Genital tract infection
Urinary tract infection
Deep vein thrombosis
Mastitis and breast engorgement
Respiratory tract infection, especially after anaesthesia
Other unrelated causes
Anaemia.

SEPSIS

Genital tract infection

Microbiology: In past: beta-haemolytic streptococci
Gp B were important.

Now: anaerobic steptococci (34%)
staphylococci (23%)
non-haemolytic steptococci (19%)
coliforms (8%)
remainder (16%)

Any part of genital tract, from vulva to ovary and including the parametrium, may become infected. Usually an ascending infection.

Features:	Malaise Lower abdominal pain Fever Tender uterus.
Management:	Appropriate antibiotic after taking swabs and blood cultures (high vaginal and cervical swab); give cephalosporin metronidazole until sensitivities known Analgesia Hydration and rest.
Complications:	Sterility Chronic pelvic inflammatory disease Broad ligament abscess Septicaemia Death.

Urinary tract infection
Common, especially following instrumentation
Often due to *Esch. coli.*

Features:	Dysuria, frequency Dull headache Pyrexia.
Investigations:	Haemoglobin, white cell count and differential Mid-stream urine High vaginal swab.
Treatment:	Rest Analgesia High fluid intake Broad spectrum antibiotic until sensitivities known Mist. pot. cit. for dysuria.

Breast infection

Predisposing factors:	Poor nipple care
	Breast engorgement.

Features:　Hot, red, tender area in breast
Usually staphylococcal
Pyrexia
Brawny swelling suggests abscess
  formation.

Management:　If caught early, i.e. less than 48 h,
  antibiotics and suppress lactation
Later (or if any suggestion of abscess)
  incision and drainage
Be aware: can express milk from infected
  side and feed from healthy side.
  Antibiotics in breast milk may give
  neonate loose stools.

THROMBOEMBOLISM

Important cause of maternal death.

Thrombosis
May occur in leg or pelvic veins.

Prevention:　Early mobilisation, especially after operative
  delivery
Wear support tights
Postnatal exercises
Treat anaemia and dehydration.

Features:　Persistent tachycardia, often
  disproportionate to any pyrexia
Calf pain and tenderness
Oedema and swelling of leg
Pelvic vein thrombosis (may be
  symptomless and signless).

Investigations:　Doppler ultrasound
Venogram
Radioisotope studies
Diagnosis is important because of future
  implications.

Management:	Raise foot of bed Apply anti-embolism stockings Encourage active movement of legs Heparinise Wafarinise for 3 months.

Embolism
Four grades of severity may be recognised:

Group A:	Sudden death
Group B:	Acute dyspnoea with or without evidence of shock
Group C:	Pleuritic pain and haemoptysis, without circulatory failure
Group D:	Shortness of breath alone.
Features:	Call to stool may precede event Giant 'a' wave in jugular venous pulse (blocked pulmonary vasculature) Powerful parasternal heave Right atrial gallop (triple heart sounds, loudest in the pulmonary area) Pleural friction rub in large infarcts.
Investigations:	Chest X-ray Electrocardiogram Perfusion scan (VQ scan) Serum enzymes Pulmonary arteriography.

Management:	Acting quickly, on suspicion alone, can save lives: do not waste time doing sophisticated tests unless they are immediately available.
	Restore circulation:
	   cardiac massage
	   emergency embolectomy if available
	   thrombolytics (e.g. urokinase)
	Give oxygen
	Pain relief — morphine 15 mg i.v.

Anicoagulate:
heparin — 25 000 units immediately
followed by 25 000 units 6 hourly
for 24 hours
warfarinise.

POSTPARTUM HAEMORRHAGE

Secondary postpartum haemorrhage

Definition: Any excess (note no specified volume)
genital tract bleeding after 24 hours from
delivery.

Causes: First few days:
retained products —
membranes + /or placenta
blood clots
Later: infection.

Features: Fresh vaginal bleeding after lochia has
turned brown
Tender bulky uterus
Os may be open
Pyrexia
Offensive discharge.

Management: Resuscitation as needed
High vaginal swab
Appropriate antibiotics
Surgical exploration (beware of perforating
the soft uterus), with evacuation of
retained products as appropriate.

PSYCHIATRIC COMPLICATIONS

Postnatal depression is common (60%)
Ranges from '5th day blues' to a severe depressive psychosis.

Features: Rejection of baby
Delusions
Confusion.

Management: Close observation
Mild antidepressants
Counselling as required
Oestrogen/progesterone therapy.

DRUGS AND BREAST FEEDING

Safe	Safety unknown	Unsafe
Heparin	Aminoglycosides	Chloramphenicol
Penicillins		Tetracyclines
Cephalosporins	Beta-blockers	Indomethacin
Codeine	Sulphonamides	Phenylbutazone
Pethidine	Oestrogens (low dose)	Oestrogen (high dose)
Paracetamol		Lithium
Methyldopa	Carbimazole	Iodides
Benzodiazepines	Thyroxine	Aspirin
Phenothiazines	Oral hypoglycaemics	
Tricyclics	Isoniazid	
Digoxin		
Insulin		
Progesterones		
Antacids		
Bulk laxatives		
Ethambutol		
Warfarin		

Maternal and perinatal mortality

MATERNAL MORTALITY

Obstetricians in England and Wales have performed their own medical audit in the form of the Confidential Enquiries into Maternal Deaths since 1952. (Scotland has been included since 1965.) The report for 1985–87 was the first combining information from the four countries of the United Kingdom. These enquiries collect detailed information about maternal deaths over a 3-year period, and thus allow identification of avoidable factors in the causes of death. It has therefore been possible to alter practice so as to considerably reduce maternal mortality. The relative importance of different causes of death has changed as a result of changes in practice brought about by the Confidential Enquiries.

An avoidable cause of death was, for example, identified in obstetric anaesthetic practice in that often inexperienced junior anaesthetists on their own were involved with cases that went wrong. The British Association of Anaesthetists recommended that two anaesthetists should be present for obstetric anaesthetics, one of whom should be experienced in obstetric anaesthesia. Another report identified an association between artificial rupture of the membranes combined with immediate stimulation of the uterus, resulting in the rare amniotic fluid embolus, which killed 14 women in England and Wales in the triennium 1972–75.

MATERNAL DEATH

Definition: A death occurring during pregnancy, during labour, or as a consequence of pregnancy within *1 year* of the delivery or abortion.

Deaths: 'True' — directly due to pregnancy
Associated — due to other causes (i.e. no causal relationship)

Selected facts from the latest report covering 1985–87 (published 1991; HMSO):	139 direct obstetric deaths (56%) 84 indirect obstetric deaths (34%) 26 fortuitous deaths (10%) Total births 2 293 508 Total maternal deaths 174 Maternal mortality 7.6 per 100 000 total births.
Main causes:	Pulmonary embolus — 32 deaths Hypertensive diseases — 27 deaths Haemorrhage — 10 deaths All other causes — 105 deaths.
All other causes:	Abortion Caesarean section Anaesthetic deaths Ruptured uterus Amniotic fluid embolus Ectopic pregnancy Puerperal sepsis Miscellaneous.

Indirect and fortuitous causes:	Cardiac disease in pregnancy (3rd cause of maternal death after PE and hypertension)
	Arterial aneurysms
	Alcoholic disorders
	Auto-immune diseases
	Blood diseases:
	    sickle cell anaemia
	    leukaemia
	Cerebral infarction
	Diabetes mellitus
	Encephalitis
	Epilepsy
	GI tract disorders
	Hepatic failure
	Intracranial haemorrhage
	Kyphoscoliosis
	Meningitis
	Cancer
	Respiratory disease
	Renal disease
	Pituitary infarction
	Suicide.

The *Report on Confidential Enquiries into Maternal Deaths in the United Kingdom 1985–87*, HMSO, London 1991, makes fascinating reading, and the authors strongly recommend that it is read by undergraduates as an adjunct to the standard textbooks.

PERINATAL MORTALITY AND MORBIDITY

Perinatal mortality is the sum of stillbirths and deaths during the first week of life, and the perinatal mortality rate is the total per 1000 births.

Between 1980 and 1989, the perinatal mortality rate fell from 13.4 per 1000 live and still-births to 8.3 per 1000. (The stillbirth rate fell from 7.3 per 1000 live and still-births to 4.7 per 1000 during the same period.)

Main causes:	Prematurity (nearly 50% of perinatal deaths occur in preterm infants)
	Intrapartum asphyxia
	Birth trauma
	Malformations
	Hyaline membrane disease
	Pneumonia
	Unknown (10%).
Associated factors:	Place of residence (S and E best)
	Maternal age (best early 20s)
	Parity (2nd baby best)
	Social class (1 best, 5 worst)
	Poor obstetric history
	Poor antenatal care
	Gestational age
	Birth weight
	PET
	Bleeding before 28 weeks
	Breech delivery
	Forceps delivery
	Prolonged labour
	Precipitate labour.

Perinatal morbidity

The incidence of perinatal morbidity is difficult to assess: what criteria are used over what time scale? Which individuals are taken as controls? There is also the difficulty of follow-up.

Perinatal morbidity includes brain damage and the effect of malformations. Although most of the factors affecting the PMR are likely in lesser degrees to influence perinatal morbidity, it is recognised that low social class (and its consequences) are a major factor in increasing perinatal morbidity.

The trend towards smaller families combined with the low PMR (which may have reached its lowest practical level) is resulting in greater emphasis on the quality of obstetric care. Thus it is appropriate to compare not only the mortality rates of different practices, such as forceps delivery and caesarean section, but also their morbidity. Roughly equal mortalities may mask differences in morbidity. At the end of the day, parents want high quality children, and it is the job of the obstetrician to ensure a healthy baby for a healthy mother.

Index